Current Approaches

Risk/Benefits of Antidepressants

Edited by
B E Leonard & S W Parker

duphar
medical relations

© 1988 Duphar Laboratories Limited

All rights reserved. No part of this publication may be reproduced, stored in a retrieval system or transmitted, in any form or by any means, electronic, mechanical, photocopying or otherwise, without the prior permission of the publisher.

First published 1988

ISBN 1-870678-05-2

Printed in Great Britain by
Inprint (Litho) Ltd., Southampton.

CONTENTS

Editor's Foreword   iv

Chairman: P K Bridges
Senior Lecturer and Consultant Psychiatrist
Guy's Hospital, London

Cost Benefit Analysis of Tricyclic Antidepressant Overdose   1
B E Leonard

Side Effects and Interactions   13
P Turner

Cognitive and Behavioural Consequences of Antidepressants   18
I Hindmarch

Antidepressants and the Elderly   25
P Crome

Discussion   32

Failure to Treat Depression   38
A W Clare

Toxicity in Overdose   44
J A Henry

Reporting the Risks   53
C Speirs

Discussion   59

List of Delegates   63

EDITOR'S FOREWORD

Suicidal ideation is a common symptom of endogenous depression and it is universally accepted that such patients are at a greater risk of self-poisoning and suicide than other members of the general population. Safety in overdosage is therefore an important feature of any drug prescribed for depressed patients. Of these, the tricyclic antidepressants are undoubtedly therapeutically effective. However, they are responsible for in excess of 350 deaths in England and Wales per annum at the present time (Proudfoot, 1986). With the increasing emphasis by the Health Authorities on the need to prescribe cheaper drugs, there is a natural tendancy for clinicians to use the effective but older tricyclic antidepressants and thereby increase the risk of killing the patient who takes an intentional overdose. This is reflected in the details of the number of fatal poisonings in England and Wales for the period 1977-1984. Thus the total number of fatal poisonings decreased by 28% (from 2966 to 2148) over this period while the percentage of deaths involving antidepressants remained constant at approximately 25% (Office of Population Censuses and Surveys 1977 - 1986). Thus despite the introduction of a number of non-tricyclic (e.g. mianserin, trazodone, fluvoxamine) and novel tricyclic (e.g. lofepramine) antidepressants for which there is now substantial evidence indicating their relative safety in overdose (see Cassidy and Henry, 1987), the number of fatalities resulting from antidepressant overdosage has changed little. This is partly due to the lack of awareness by clinicians of the toxicity of the older tricyclic drugs and partly because the cost of the course of treatment is often emphasized at the expense of safety. Even the legislative authorities would appear to place more emphasis on the rare idiosynchratic adverse effects of such newer antidepressants as nomifensine or zimeldine than on the well established toxicity of the older tricyclics. This is not an argument against careful monitoring of adverse effects of new drugs but rather an emphasis on the need to carefully balance efficacy with safety considerations for all drugs, old and new. Thus a cost; benefit analysis of any antidepressant must take into account

a) the risk to the patient in not treating the depression
b) the benefits of treating the patient with an antidepressant and
c) the risks of adverse effects of the antidepressant as a consequence of treatment.

It is not the intention of these brief Editorial remarks to summarize the main points raised by the various authors in this volume, but rather to give a background to the Symposium which was held in September 1987 at the Royal Society, London, to critically discuss the various issues involved in assessing the cost: benefit analysis of antidepressants. It is hoped that this publication, will extend beyond the specialist pharmacologist and clinical toxicologist to reach practising clinicians who are responsible for prescribing the bulk of antidepressants. The aim of this publication is to present a broad and balanced view of the "state of the art" regarding antidepressant toxicity for which the practising clinician can objectively draw his or her own conclusions regarding the cost of the drug versus the benefit to the patients. In the last analysis only the mortality rate for antidepressant overdosage will suggest whether such intentions have been realized!

I would like to conclude by thanking Dr. Susan Parker and her colleagues at Duphar Laboratories for their prompt and efficient editorial assistance which has enabled the Symposium to be printed in less than six months.

B E Leonard
Professor of Pharmacology
University College, Galway, Republic of Ireland

References

1. Cassidy, S. and Henry, J. (1987). Fatal toxicity of antidepressant drugs in overdosage. BMJ., 295, 1021 - 1024.

2. Proudfoot, A.J. (1986). Acute poisoning with antidepressants and lithium. Prescribers Journal 26, 97 - 106.

COST BENEFIT ANALYSIS OF TRICYCLIC ANTIDEPRESSANT OVERDOSAGE

B.E. Leonard
Professor of Pharmacology
University College, Galway, Republic of Ireland.

Toxicity of Antidepressants Following Overdose

Suicidal thoughts are frequently experienced by the depressed patient which predisposes such a patient to a greater risk of self-poisoning and suicide than other members of the general population.Safety in overdosage is therefore an important attribute of any drug, particularly antidepressants, which are prescribed to treat the symptoms of depression. Despite the introduction of a number of novel "second generation" antidepressants during the last ten years, tricyclic antidepressants are still the most widely used and, as such, most commonly encountered in antidepressant overdosage. It has been estimated that the tricyclic antidepressants comprise the single most important group of drugs causing serious CNS depression in the U.K. and, in recent years, have been responsible for the deaths of approximately 350 persons per year in England and Wales alone (Proudfoot, 1986). There is evidence that the incidence of antidepressant overdosage is increasing at least in some parts of the British Isles. Thus McAleer et al. (1986) have reported that in some centres in Northern Ireland, the incidence of antidepressant overdosage increased from 19% of all poisoning cases admitted to the intensive care units in 1973 - 1977 to 26% in the period 1978 - 1983. By contrast, Crome and Newman (1979) found that the number of fatalities due to tricyclic antidepressant overdosage was approximately 12% of the total fatalities due to drug overdosage in 1975, but remained fairly constant, at approximately 14% of total fatalities due to drug overdosage, for the period 1977 - 1984 (OPCS quoted by Montgomery and Pinder, 1987). Thus despite the introduction of novel antidepressants, which appear to be safer in overdosage than the standard tricyclic drugs, there is little evidence to suggest that the magnitude of the problem has changed appreciably in the last ten years. A somewhat similar situation is emerging in the United States of America where tricyclic antidepressant overdosage is the third most common cause of drug related death (U.S. Department of Health and Human Services, 1983). However, it should be emphasized that apart from trazodone, loxapine and the monoamine oxidase inhibitors only the standard tricyclic antidepressants, such as amitriptyline and imipramine, are available in the United States.

Only the United Kingdom publishes annually detailed figures of the number of fatalities following self-poisoning whether intentional or accidental. From such statistics it is possible to compare the relative toxicity of non-tricyclic with tricyclic antidepressants. The latest figures from England and Wales for four commonly prescribed tricyclic antidepressants compared with the tetracyclic antidepressant mianserin are shown in Table I (OPCS, 1985).

Table I
Deaths from poisoning by antidepressants (1985)

Drug	Accidental Poisoning	Suicide	Undetermined	Total
Amitriptyline	11 (5)	52 (5)	14 (3)	77 (13)
Dothiepin	3 (1)	58 (3)	21 (3)	87 (7)
Imipramine	1	12	7	20
Trimipramine	2 (1)	7 (1)	3	12 (2)
Mianserin	—	5 (1)	1	6 (1)

Figures in parenthesis suggest numbers of patients having taken the antidepressant with alcohol. (Figures are for single drugs alone).

Mianserin was chosen as a representative non-tricyclic antidepressant as it has been marketed in the U.K. for approximately ten years and therefore a reasonably large population of depressed patients would have been exposed to the drug to allow comparison to be made between its toxicity and those of the standard tricyclic antidepressants as shown in Table I.

A truer representation of the relative toxicity of the antidepressants in common use in Northern Europe and North America is obtained when the number of fatalities is expressed in terms of the prescriptions issued. Such an analysis has recently been published by Montgomery and Pinder (1987) which substantially replicates that presented by Leonard (1986). This is summarized in Table II together with an estimate of the number of patients treated with the antidepressants in England and Wales for the period 1977 - 1984.

There is no satisfactory method of accurately calculating the fatalities per million patients treated as the data relating to the precise number of patients treated with these antidepressants over the seven year period is unknown. Nevertheless, an estimate has been made based on the total sales of the respective antidepressants in kg (IMS) divided by an average dose and duration of treatment. For the tricyclic antidepressants, an average daily dose of 112.5 mg was used and for mianserin the value was 45 mg. In all cases, the duration of treatment was taken to be 60 days. This method of calculation has been cited by Montgomery and Pinder (1987) and Leonard (1986).

Table II
Estimated incidence of death from overdose of antidepressants in England and Wales for the period 1977 - 1984.

Drug	Estimated No. patients treated (millions)	No. fatalities Single drug	No. fatalities Multiple drugs	Single drug fatalities per million patients
Amitriptyline	4.8	808	447	168
Dothiepin	3.1	453	159	145
Imipramine	1.8	201	102	111
Doxepin	0.6	67	42	111
Maprotiline	0.5	60	24	120
Trimipramine	1.2	109	85	90
Clomipramine	1.0	34	35	34
Mianserin	2.0	27	53	13

The number of fatalities include all patients who died irrespective of whether the overdosage was intentional or accidental. (Figures obtained from the publications of the Office of Population Censuses and Surveys for the period 1977 - 1984).

The relative incidence of fatalities from antidepressant overdosage may be calculated from the cumulative figures for the period 1977-1984 from England and Wales by expressing the ratio of the percentage of fatalities for each antidepressant to the percentage of patients treated with that antidepressant over the same time period. The results from such calculations are shown in Table III.

Table III
Relative incidence of deaths from overdose of some commonly used antidepressants (After Jenner : unpublished)

Drug	% Patients treated	% Total fatalities	Relative indices of death
Amitriptyline	31.5	45.9	1.46
Dothiepin	20.4	25.7	1.26
Imipramine	12.2	11.4	0.93
Doxepin	4.1	3.8	0.93
Maprotiline	3.7	3.4	0.91
Trimipramine	8.0	6.2	0.77
Clomipramine	6.8	1.9	0.28
Mianserin	12.9	1.5	0.12

The results of these analyses clearly indicate that the most widely used tricyclic antidepressants are also the most toxic in overdose and that the newer antidepressants that have been widely prescribed for many years are less toxic. Of the other second generation antidepressants that have also been available for a number of years, trazodone and nomifensine have been the subject of detailed investigations. Thus Ali and Crome (1984) found that of the 74 patients having taken an overdose of nomifensine, either alone or in combination with other drugs over the period 1977 - 1983, no deaths occurred, the most common symptom shown was drowsiness. Regarding trazodone, drowsiness, dizziness and nausea appear to be the most common features when this drug is taken in excess but there is no evidence that the drug is fatal (Proudfoot, 1986). Of the remaining second generation antidepressants that has been available since 1977, 4 deaths have been reported following the ingestion of high doses of viloxazine but, in general, it would appear that this drug is safer than the conventional tricyclic antidepressants (Proudfoot, 1986). Of the tricyclic antidepressants that have been introduced in the last five years, lofepramine would appear to be unique in that no cases of fatalities have so far been reported, following ingestion of this drug alone, either in the U.K. or Scandinavia. Thus Heath (1984) reviewed 20 cases of lofepramine overdose reported in Sweden and reported that all survived. The incidence of those patients exhibiting severe coma (Grade 3 or 4), sinus tachycardia and respiratory depression requiring artificial respiration after taking an overdose of lofepramine was much reduced compared to those taking an equivalent quantity of a standard tricyclic antidepressant such as amitriptyline. In the U.K. Proudfoot (1986) found that of 20 patients having taken an overdose of lofepramine, 4 were in coma and only 1 of these required assisted ventilation. It would therefore appear that, despite its tricyclic structure, lofepramine is less toxic than the older members of the tricyclic antidepressant series and should be considered along with the newer second generation drugs. The reason for the apparent safety of lofepramine is uncertain despite the well established fact that it is partly metabolized to the tricyclic antidepressant desipramine *in vivo;* Leonard (1987) has reviewed the pharmacological profile and the possible explanations for its relatively low toxicity.

Of the most recently introduced novel antidepressants in the U.K., the serotonin uptake inhibitor fluvoxamine would so far appear not to have caused any deaths in overdose; to date some 30 patients have attempted suicide unsuccessfully (Benfield and Ward, 1986).

It may be concluded that with the possible exception of clomipramine, all the standard tricyclic antidepressants are relatively toxic in overdose and there is little evidence to suggest that any one drug in current use is superior to any other. Furthermore there would appear to be no relationship between the presumed selectivity in the ability of the tricyclic antidepressant to inhibit the re-uptake of noradrenaline or serotonin and its toxicity. Thus dothiepin is a moderately selective serotonin re-uptake inhibitor, while amitriptyline is approximately equi-active in inhibiting both noradrenaline and serotonin re-uptake; these drugs occupy the first two positions in the toxicity table for antidepressant fatalities. Conversely maprotiline is a potent and selective noradrenaline re-uptake inhibitor while imipramine shows slight preference for inhibiting serotonion re-uptake; these drugs are equally toxic in overdose. Thus it seems unlikely that there is any direct relationship between the effects of antidepressants on those biogenic amine neurotransmitters that are presumed to be malfunctioning in the depressed patient and their toxicity on overdose. Presumably the toxicity of the tricyclic antidepressants in particular is associated with their anticholinergic effects, α_1-adrenoceptor antagonistic effects or, more particularly, their membrane stabilizing (quinidine-like) effects which may become prominent following overdose (Callaham, 1979).

Cost: Benefit Analysis of Antidepressants.

Three criteria must be applied when attempting to undertake such analysis.
a) The risk to the patient in not treating the depression
b) The benefits of treating the depressed patient with antidepressants and
c) The risks of adverse effects of the antidepressants as a consequence of treatment.

a) Risk of Not Treating the Patient

Suicidal thoughts are an integral part of depression and one of the most serious aspects of depressive illness is the number of patients who commit suicide. This has been estimated to be as high as 15% in some studies (Guse and Robins, 1970). Thus the greatest risk is failure by the clinician to provide adequate treatment for patients who could benefit from it, the consequences ranging from an unnecessary prolongation of the illness to a possible fatal outcome. Any statistics relating to the duration of illness or incidence of suicide that may occur if the patient is not adequately treated do not take into account the devastating effect of the illness on the quality of life of the patient and the patient's family. Elderly patients are particularly vulnerable not only because of the increased incidence of the illness in this age group but also because of the increase in significant life events (e.g. physical illness, death of a spouse) which may exacerbate the illness (Murphy, 1985). Murphy's study suggests a rather poor overall prognosis for depression in the elderly with nearly 66% of the patients investigated being unchanged, deteriorated further or dead within one year of diagnosis. Not all psychogeriatricians would favour such a pessimistic view however (Wattis, 1986). It is therefore self-evident that treatment of the depressed patient is essential and as some patients, variously estimated to be between 3% and 50% according to the study of Kresser-Hermsdorf et al. (1985), attempt suicide on these drugs, care must be taken in the selection of potentially toxic drugs for the treatment of the condition. Thus any assessment of the advantages of a particular antidepressant must take into account a risk/benefit analysis of potential toxicity in overdose.

b) Benefits of Treatment with Antidepressants.

The most obvious benefit of antidepressant therapy lies in the relief of the symptoms thereby reducing the risk of suicide, improving the quality of life of the patient and increasing the life expectancy.

Estimates of the level of efficacy of the standard tricyclic antidepressants vary but systematic reviews of controlled clinical trials indicate that these drugs are superior to placebo in 60 - 70% of all studies (Gerner et al., 1980). It is also important to note that there is no unequivocal evidence to suggest that any antidepressant is superior to a standard tricyclic such as amitriptyline either in terms of efficacy or speed of onset of antidepressant response. Most clinicians would agree with the view that one third of hospitalized depressed patients respond well to tricyclic medication, one third have a moderate response while the remainder respond poorly; approximately 20% of all patients fail to respond to a course of a single tricyclic antidepressant (Montgomery, 1986).

In most studies of the efficacy of antidepressant therapy, the placebo response rate has been estimated to be of the order of 30% (Burrows et al., 1976).

Despite the evidence from studies that some of the new antidepressants with serotonin re-uptake inhibitory properties show an earlier onset in the reduction of anxiety symptoms and suicidal ideation (Ofsti, 1982; Feldmann and Denber, 1982), there is little evidence to suggest that the newer antidepressants which are highly selective for inhibiting the re-uptake of either noradrenaline or serotonin have any therapeutic advantage over the nonspecific 'standard' tricyclics (see Montgomery, 1982). The major advantage of the second generation antidepressants over the standard tricyclics lies in their reduced incidence of side effects and comparative safety in overdosage.

In these days of economic restraint, the case is often made by Health Authorities that the relatively low cost of the older tricyclic antidepressants should be considered a benefit. However as Henry and Martin (1987) have remarked, the cost of a course of treatment should only be used as a basis for choosing between drugs once it has been shown that there is no significant clinical difference either in terms of efficacy or side effect profile between them. As has been indicated elsewhere in this review, it is clear that all of the older tricyclic antidepressants are toxic in overdose and have a higher incidence of side effects than the newer antidepressants. It would seem morally indefensible to argue that the unit cost of an antidepressant should be the major criterion for selecting it. Safety and a reduced incidence of adverse effect should form part of the equation, as well as efficacy, when a cost benefit analysis of antidepressant treatment is made.

c) Risk of Adverse Effects of Antidepressant Treatment.

The major adverse effects of all of the older tricyclic antidepressant drugs is their anticholinergic activity (blurred vision, dry mouth, difficulty in micturition, constipation, tachycardia). Johnson (1983) has studied the reason for non-compliance amongst non-hospital patients being treated with antidepressants and showed that only 46% of patients being treated with the older tricyclic drugs showed compliance compared to 71% taking one of the newer non-tricyclic drugs. The majority of the patients discontinued taking their antidepressants when they experienced side effects, the symptoms most poorly tolerated being sedation and a dry mouth. Johnson (1986) has also stressed the importance of doctor-patient communication in ensuring that optimal compliance is achieved as the majority of patients surveyed in a large general practitioner based study seemed to obtain their information on psychotropic drug medication from the media and not from their family doctor or any other informed medical source.

While the older tricyclic antidepressants vary in their anticholinergic side effects (amitriptyline and imipramine being the most potent, followed by dothiepin, doxepin and clomipramine with desipramine and the new tricyclic lofepramine being the least potent), the monoamine oxidase inhibitors and the second generation drugs (with the exception of maprotiline which should be considered to be a modified tricyclic compound) have little anticholinergic activity in therapeutic doses. Henry and Martin (1987) have recently summarized the relative incidence of the anticholinergic side effects of the various antidepressants.

The adverse effects of tricyclic antidepressants on the cardiovascular system are well established. Such effects, in therapeutic doses, range from postural hypotension due to adrenoceptor antagonism, to tachycardia. Some investigators have suggested that there is an increased mortality in patients taking tricyclic antidepressants due primarily to the decreased myocardial contractility which these drugs are shown to cause under experimental conditions (Coull et al., 1978; Moir et al., 1972; 1973). More recent studies (Veith et al., 1982; Burrows et al., 1976) have suggested however that such quinidine-like effects of the older tricyclic drugs are of little clinical consequences in patients with cardiac defects (apart from those with intra-ventricular conduction disorders: Roos, 1983). It is of interest that the second generation antidepressant trazodone has been shown to exacerbate cardiac arrhythmias in patients predisposed to the condition (Janowsky et al., 1983; Himmeehoch et al., 1984), an effect that does not appear to be due to a quinidine-like property of the molecule. While the adverse cardiac effects of the older tricyclic antidepressants would not appear to be of major significance after therapeutic doses, arrhythmias and depression of myocardial contractility appear to be the principal causes of death following overdose of these drugs (Pentel and Benowitz, 1986). When assessing the risk-benefit ratio of not treating depressed patient with an antidepressant, it is also important to take into account the suggestion that the overall mortality due to cardiac disease may be higher in untreated depressed patients than those being treated with drugs or ECT (Avery and Winokur, 1976). Clearly special attention should be given to elderly depressives whose susceptibility to the adverse effects of antidepressants is greater than those in younger age groups (Gerner, 1985; Davies et al., 1971); particularly as these patients are more prone to cardiovascular disease. In addition, elderly patients are more likely to be taking other types of medication so that drug interactions are liable to play a more significant role in the management of their depressive illness. Drugs with minimal anticholinergic activity, such as mianserin, trazodone, fluvoxamine, lofepramine or monoamine oxidase inhibitors should therefore receive particular attention when considering the treatment of elderly depressed patients.

In addition to their antidepressant properties, most antidepressants have CNS effects which may be considered to be disadvantageous to the patient. The older tricyclics, and several of the second generation drugs such as mianserin and trazodone, are histamine type 1 receptor antagonists which probably accounts for their sedative effects. This often results in daytime drowsiness which is a frequent reason for administering these drugs as a single daily dose at night. Nomifensine, recently withdrawn world-wide because of some fatal hypersensitivity reactions, had a stimulant effect while many of the recently developed specific serotonin re-uptake inhibitors such as fluvoxamine (Saletu et al., 1983) have slight alerting effects at therapeutic doses. The monoamine oxidase inhibitors may also cause CNS stimulation, particularly drugs such as tranylcypromine which have amphetamine-like effects. Many tricyclic antidepressants are pro-convulsive in both therapeutic doses and in overdose (Proudfoot, 1986); the modified tricyclic antidepressant maprotiline has been reported to provoke convulsions in non-epileptic patients (Jabbari et al., 1985). In general, the second generation antidepressants do not appear to exhibit it pro-convulsive activity, neither do the monoamine oxidase inhibitors.

A frequently reported adverse effect following prolonged antidepressant medication is change in body weight. This can occur as a consequence of an improvement in appetite following the reduction of the depressive symptoms. However, the older tricyclic antidepressants may cause a craving for high carbohyrdrate foods leading to an excessive weight gain; amitriptyline is particularly hazardous in this respect (Paykel et al., 1973) and the monoamine oxidase inhibitors have also been reported to have these adverse effects (Rabkin et al., 1985). Most of the newer antidepressants, in particular those like fluvoxamine and fluoxetine, would not appear to adversely affect the body weight of patients undergoing treatment (Benfield and Ward, 1986). Nausea, occasional vomiting and headache are the most frequent side effects reported to occur with such specific serotonin uptake inhibitors as fluvoxamine and fluoxetine.

In addition to the well established adverse effects of antidepressants, unpredictable adverse effects may occasionally occur which may be more correctly considered to be idiosynchratic reactions. Thus tricyclic antidepressants have been rarely reported to produce cholestatic jaundice, rashes, urticaria and vasculitis while with the second generation antidepressants priapism has been reported to occur with trazodone (Scher et al., 1983) and bone marrow depression, exhibiting as agranulocytotic granulocytopaenia, has been reported to occur following mianserin; this effect would appear to be more common in elderly patients (CSM, 1985).

Monitoring Antidepressants for Adverse Effects

While the potential efficacy and adverse effects of a new antidepressant will to some extent be predicted shortly after its registration, the toxicity in overdose can only be assessed after the drug has been widely used for several years. Drug monitoring is clearly very important in assessing not only the toxicity but also the serious side effects which may arise following the extensive use of any drug. A major problem arises in assessing the significance of rare, but serious, side effects particularly when one takes into account the relative toxicity of the older tricyclic antidepressants in overdose. Lewis (1981) has calculated that if any adverse side effect occurs in 1 : 10,000 patients, 65,000 patients must be treated with the drug in order for three cases of that adverse effect to occur. In practise, patients exhibiting serious side effects are likely to be taking other types of medication which may make the casual relationship between the new drug and the adverse effect difficult to assess. Furthermore, the frequency of the side effects may be increased by the age of the patient (cf. blood dyscrasias following mianserin administration) and by such factors as physical ill health. Thus there is invariably a considerable delay before the adverse effect of a new antidepressant may be unequivocally established. The aim of post-marketing surveillance is to alert the medical profession to the probability of such side effects occurring. In the U.K. and Republic of Ireland, a "yellow card" system has been implemented by the Committee for the Safety of Medicines and the National Drugs Advisory Board respectively, in an attempt to obtain such data. However it is doubtful whether the returns from such surveys of new drugs accurately reflect the extent of adverse effects. One of the main reasons for this lies in the preferential reporting of data on adverse effects. For example, clinicians know that the older antidepressants cause dry mouth, blurred vision, etc. and that at least 17 different classes of drugs (varying from sulphonamides, diuretics and antiarrhythmic drugs to phenothiazines and anticonvulsants) are likely to cause leucopenia and other types of blood dyscrasia. Unless an unexpected death occurs in a patient on such medication, such adverse effects are less likely to be reported than if a patient is being treated with a newly marketed drug whose side effects are likely to receive greater attention. This is not an argument against the use of surveillance procedures but does serve to emphasize the incomplete nature of the adverse effects data due to preferential reporting, or under-reporting in the case of well established drugs, which makes an assessment of the risk-benefit ratio for a new drug difficult to obtain. An additional complication may arise regarding the evaluation of the effects of interacting medication on the frequency of side effects of the new drug. Clearly there is a need for a more thorough and objective mechanism whereby post-marketing surveillance maybe undertaken by the Health Authorities.

Conclusion

In addition to the efficacy of an antidepressant, the following factors must be taken into account when undertaking a cost benefit analysis of such a drug:

a) the frequency of non-fatal side effects which may limit patient compliance,
b) the frequency of unpredictable serious side effects (e.g. blood dyscrasias),
c) the incidence of fatalities following intentional or accidental overdose,
d) the incidence of side effects related to the age of the patient. As the incidence of depression is higher in the elderly, who as a group are more likely to suffer physical ill health for which other types of medication is often required, particular care must be taken to assess the side effects of a new antidepressant in this age group,
e) the unit cost of antidepressant treatment. This should be considered only after all other factors mentioned above have been taken into consideration.

Using these criteria, there would appear to be every reason for considering the replacement of the older tricyclic antidepressants with the newer non-tricyclic drugs in the first line treatment of depression, unless of course, the unit cost of treatment is the only consideration!

Acknowledgements

I wish to express my gratitude to the many colleagues for the fruitful discussions on this subject which have helped to lay the basis of this article. In particular, I am most grateful to Drs. Paul Jenner, John Henry, Roger Pinder and Mr. Mervyn Whitford for sources of information on adverse effects and antidepressant overdose.

References

1. Ali, C. and Crome, P. (1984). The clinical toxicology of nomifensine: an update. Roy. Soc. Med. Int. Cong. and Symp. Ser. No. 70. 121 - 123.
2. Avery, D. and Winokur, G. (1976). Mortality in depressed patients treated with electroconvulsive therapy and antidepressants. Arch. Gen. Psychiat., *33*, 1029.
3. Benfield, P. and Ward, A. (1986) Fluvoxamine : a review of its pharmacodynamic and pharmacokinetic properties and therapeutic efficacy in depressive illness. Drugs *32*, 313 - 334.
4. Burrows, G.D., Vohra, J. and Hurst, D. (1976). Cardiac effects of different tricyclic antidepressant drugs. Br. J. Psychiat., *129*, 335 - 341.
5. Callaham, M. (1979) Tricyclic antidepressant overdose. JACEP *8*, 413 - 425.
6. Committee for the Safety of Medicines, Update (1985). Adverse reactions to antidepressants. Br. Med. J. *291*, 1638.
7. Crome, P. and Newman, B. (1979) Fatal tricyclic antidepressant poisoning J. Roy. Soc. Med *72*, 649 - 653.
8. Coull, D.C., Crooks, J., Dingwall-Fordyce, I., Scott, A.M. and Weir, R.D. (1970) Amitriptyline and cardiac disease : risk of sudden death identified by monitoring system. Lancet, *II*, 590 - 591.

9. Davies, R.K., Tucker, D.J., Harrow, M. and Detre, J.P. (1971). Confusional episodes and antidepressant medication. Amer. J. Psychiat., *128*, 127.
10. Feldmann, H.S. and Denber, H.C.B. (1982). Long-term study of fluvoxamine : a new rapid-acting antidepressant. Int. Pharmacopsychiat., *17*, 114 - 122.
11. Gerner, R.H. (1985). Present status of drug therapy of depression in late life. J. Affect. Dis., Suppl 1., S23 - S31.
12. Gerner, R.H., Eastbrook, W., Stever, J. and Jarvik, L. (1980). Treatment of geriatric depression with trazodone, imipramine and placebo - a double-blind study. J. Clin. Psychiat., *41*, 216 - 220.
13. Guse, S.B. and Robins, E. (1970). Suicide among primary affective disorders. Br. J. Psychiat., *117*, 437 - 438.
14. Heath, A. (1984) Suicidal overdoses of antidepressants with special reference to lofepramine. Int. Med., Suppl. *10:* 27 - 30.
15. Henry, J.A. and Martin, A.J. (1987). The risk-benefit assessment of antidepressant drugs. Medical Toxicology, *2*, 445 - 462.
16. Himmelhoch, M.J., Schechtman, K. and Auchenback, R. (1984). The role of trazodone in the treatment of depressed cardiac patients. Psychopathol., *17*, Suppl. 2, 51 - 63.
17. Jabbari, B., Bryan, G., Mars Lee and Gunderson, C.H. (1985). Incidence of seizure with tricyclic and tetracyclic antidepressants. Arch. Neurol., *42*, 480 - 481.
18. Janowsky, D., Curtis, G. and Zisook, S. (1983). Ventricular arrhythmias possibly aggravated by trazodone. Am.J. Psychiat., *140*, 796 - 797.
19. Jenner, P. (Personal Communication).
20. Johnson, D.A.W. (1983). Depression : treatment compliance in general practise. Acta Psychiat. Scand., *63* (Suppl. 290), 447 - 453.
21. Johnson, D.A.W. (1986). Non-compliance with antidepressant therapy - an underestimated problem. Int. Med., Suppl. *11:* 14 - 17.
22. Kresser-Hermsdorf, M., Muller-Oerlinghausen, B. and Ibe, K. (1985). Poisoning with antidepressive drugs : a five year restrospective study. Int.J. Clin. Pharmac. Ther. Toxicol., *23*, 540 - 547.
23. Leonard, B.E. (1986). Toxicity of antidepressants. Lancet *IV*, 1105.
24. Leonard, B.E. (1987). A comparison of the pharmacological properties of the novel tricyclic antidepressant lofepramine with its major metabolite desipramine : a review. Int. Clin. Psychopharmac. (In press).
25. Lewis, J.A. (1981). Post marketing surveillance : how many patients? TIPS *2*, 93 - 94.
26. McAleer, J.J.A., Murphy, G.J.J., Taylor, R.J., Moran, J.L.C. and O'Connor, F.A. (1986). Trends in the severity of self-poisoning. J. Roy. Soc. Med., *79*, 74 - 75.
27. Moir, D.C., Crooks, T. and Cornwell, W.B. (1972). Cardiotoxicity of amitriptyline. Lancet, *ii*, 561 - 564.
28. Moir, D.C., Dingwall-Fordyce, I. and Weir, R.D. (1973). Medicines evaluation and monitoring group : a follow-up study of cardiac patients receiving amitriptyline. Br. J. Psychiat., *134*, 382 - 389.
29. Montgomery, S.A. (1982). The non-selective aeffect of selective antidepressants. Adv. Biochem. Psychopharmac., *31*, 49 - 56.
30. Montgomery, S.A. (1986). Chemotherapy of affective disorders : future prospects. Int. Med., Suppl. *11*, 30 - 32.
31. Montgomery, S.A. and Pinder, R.M. (1987). Do some antidepressants promote suicide? Psychopharmac. *92*. 265 - 266.
32. Murphy, E. (1985). General management of depression in late life. J. Affect. Dis., Suppl. *1:* S7 - S10.
33. Ofsti, E. (1982). Citalopram - a specific 5-HT reuptake inhibitor - as an antidepressant drug : a phase II multicentre trial. Prog. Neuro-Psychopharm. Biol. Psychiat., *6*, 327 - 335.

34. Office of Population Censuses and Surveys (1985). Deaths from poisoning by solid or liquid substances : accidental, suicidal and undetermined whether accidentally taken or purposely inflicted. HMSO Series DH4 No. 11 Table 10.

35. Paykel, E.S., Mueller, P.S. and De La Vesgne, P.M. (1973). Amitriptyline, weight gain and carbohydrate craving : a side effect. Br. J. Psychiat., *123*, 501 - 507.

36. Pentel, P.R. and Benowitz, N.L. (1986). Tricyclic antidepressant poisoning : management of arrhythmias. Med. Toxicol., *1*, 101 - 121.

37. Proudfoot, A.J. (1986). Acute poisoning with antidepressants and lithium. Prescribers Journal *26*, 97 - 106.

38. Rabkin, J.G., Quitkin, F.M. and McGrath, P. (1985). Adverse reactions to monoamine oxidase inhibitors. Part II : Treatment correlates and clinical management. J. Clin. Psycopharmac., *5*, 1 - 9.

39. Roos, J.C. (1983). Cardiac effects of antidepressant drugs. A comparison of the tricyclic antidepressants and fluvoxamine. Br.J. Clin. Pharmac., *15*, S439 - S445.

40. Saletu, B., Grunberger, J. and Rajna, P. (1983). Pharmaco-EEG profiles of antidepressants. Pharmacodynamic studies with fluvoxamine. Br. J. Clin. Pharmac., *15*, (Suppl.3) S369 - S384.

41. Scher, M., Krieger, J.M. and Juergens, S. (1983) Trazodone and priapism. Am. J. Psychiat., *140*, 1362 - 1363.

42. U.S. Department of Health and Human Services, National Institute of Drug Abuse : Annual Data Report 1982. Data from the Drug Abuse Warning Network (DAWN) Series, No. 2 (1983).

43. Veith, R.C. Raskind, M. and Caldwell, H.H. (1982). Cardiovascular effects of tricyclic antidepressants in depressed patients with chronic heart disease. N. Eng. J. Med., *306*, 954 - 959.

44. Wattis, J.P. (1986) Treating depression in old people. Int. Med., Suppl. *11*, 10 - 13.

SIDE EFFECTS AND INTERACTIONS

P Turner
Professor of Pharmacology
St Bartholomew's Hospital, London

For the clinical pharmacologist antidepressant drugs are just another group of drugs. They are chemicals which interact with the body system and other drugs and there is nothing very peculiar about them as a class of compound.

We know very little about the biochemical basis of depression so we still base our teaching on the monoamine theory which is a convenient model for students to remember drugs by. We teach them that it is useful to give precursors to the monoamines but I do not propose to deal with either levodopa or tryptophan here.

It is customary to divide adverse drug reactions (ADRs) into three groups:-

i) dose-dependent adverse effects

ii) dose-independent effects

iii) pseudo-allergic effects

This last group is included for completeness, being not particularly relevant to antidepressant drugs. They include histamine mediated effects which mimic allergic reactions including urticaria and respiratory obstruction but without involving complement or antibody production.

Dose-dependent effects occur with any drug if given in sufficient quantity. Previous exposure is not a prerequisite for the reaction to occur and the treatment is to reduce the dose. This aspect is of particular relevance in treating the elderly patient.

Dose-independent effects refer to such reactions as the nomifensine-induced anaemia and haemolytic problems. They do not occur in all patients, they do not occur necessarily with all drugs, and previous exposure is generally necessary either to the drug itself or one that shares cross-antigenicity with it. Treatment consists of stopping the drug or, in the case of drugs that are not really necessary, withdrawing them from the market.

Pharmacokinetic Mechanisms Underlying ADRs

These are mechanisms that involve, to some extent, drug metabolism. We should bear in mind that very often the drugs we use are pro-drugs and what we are actually seeing in the patient is not the effect of the drug but the effect of its major metabolites. This underlies the problems involved in interpreting animal research and isolated tissue research where the parent drug used may not accurately reproduce the active principle in man. I am currently looking at a new antidepressant from

France which, when given intravenously, disappears totally from the body after thirty minutes and yet is an effective antidepressant. Its action is due to some metabolite which has not yet been isolated. Until we can identify and test the metabolite involved we are working at a very great disadvantage.

Much of the so-called specificity of the antidepressant drugs on certain monoamines disappears when the action of the metabolites is taken into account. Imipramine, for example, is itself very active on the 5-HT system but its major metabolite happens to be very much more active on the dopaminergic or noradrenergic systems. Whether this actually matters is another subject altogether.

What is important is that the phase I metabolite of a drug is usually the one which is more reactive as far as its adverse effects are concerned. Furthermore, if you have a very reactive metabolite it can interact with DNA to become carcinogenic. None of the antidepressant drugs that are on the market at the moment have any evidence of carcinogenicity. A metabolite can react with RNA or some other protein to produce cell necrosis or an LE type of phenomenon which is an important mechanism in one drug to be discussed later. Another mode of action is seen with nomifensine which produces a hapten capable of causing an allergic reaction.

Polymorphism
1. Oxidation
Patients fall into various groups according to the rate at which they metabolise drugs which means that phase I metabolites may accumulate more rapidly in some patients than in others. One form of this so-called polymorphism is in the area of oxidation of the drug. Debrisoquine has been used as a marker to characterise slow oxidators who thereby accumulate higher plasma drug levels and are unwittingly exposed to the dangers of toxicity. There are several drugs which show this phase I polymorphism involving oxidation including perhexiline and phenformin. Nortriptyline, one of the metabolites of amitriptyline, is an antidepressant which is subject to this polymorphism.

2. Enzyme Induction
Drugs that are metabolised in the liver by oxidation are also likely to be involved in drug interactions with enzyme inducers. This will be a familiar interaction to those who were practising medicine in the days before benzodiazepines were widely available when, for example, a patient with a myocardial infarction might be given a barbiturate to alleviate their anxiety. If the barbiturate was then withdrawn it was often noted that their warfarin levels would rise. The barbiturate had induced liver enzymes which in turn increased the rate of metabolism of warfarin.

Barbiturates are no longer widely used but there are other drugs which are enzyme inducers. The important interactions to note are those of the anticonvulsants (phenytoin, carbamezepine) and the antitubercular drug (rifampicin) which can increase the metabolism of tricyclic antidepressants.

Enzyme induction also occurs in people who smoke, mild and moderate alcoholics and those exposed to a range of environmental chemicals such as pesticides, polycyclic aromatic hydrocarbons and the carbon encrusted surface of barbecued meat.

Enzyme induction thus modifies the metabolism of tricyclics and it is perhaps not surprising, therefore, to find that in patients on a fixed dose of amitriptyline their actual plasma levels can vary by as much as two hundred fold. In the final analysis this polymorphism of metabolism with its genetic and environmental components may be the most important factor in determining plasma levels and thereby variation in response to antidepressants.

3. Acetylation

Another form of metabolism which is important is acetylation. This first arose with the sulphonamides, procainamide and hydralazine but also occurs with the MAOI, phenelzine. Steady state plasma levels of phenelzine in a population on a fixed dose will show two peaks. Most people, the fast acetylators, will have low plasma levels but another group will be identified who have higher levels because they are acetylating the drug more slowly and the drug is excreted more slowly. It is these patients, the slow acetylators, who do best with phenelzine because they get rid of the drug less quickly and they find it more effective but at the same time they are the patients who are going to run the risk of the cell necrosis factor. They are the ones who are going to get positive lupus tests and show the LE phonomenon.

Effects of Disease on Drug Metabolism

Disease itself can influence the metabolism of drugs. The toxicity of lithium, for example, increases in patients with renal disease and cardiac failure because they have reduced renal excretion. To make matters worse, lithium is also made more toxic in patients who are on sodium-losing diuretics.

Adverse Effects of Monoamine Oxidase Inhibitors (MAOIs)

The enzyme monoamine oxidase within the cell normally breaks down the cytoplasmic monoamines and if it is inhibited then the levels of monoamine rise within the cell and can be released. This sequence of events can be demonstrated easily using the pupil and comparing its reaction to the directly acting amine, phenylephrine, and the indirectly acting amines, tyramine and hydroxyamphetamine, in patients treated with an MAOI such as phenelzine.

The pupil responses to tyramine and hydroxyamphetamine are massive in patients receiving the MAOI compared with untreated controls, whereas the directly acting phenylephrine that does not have to release the monoamine but goes straight to the receptor, has the same effect in both groups of patients. We also know from experience that indirectly acting amines such as tyramine and phenylpropanolamine will produce a much greater rise in blood pressure in patients than in controls.

Phenylpropanolamine merits further comment because there is a lot of it around especially in medicines that are bought over the counter in pharmacies, for treating upper respiratory tract infections. It acts as a vasoconstricter and bronchodilator. Many people want to see it introduced as an OTC preparation for appetite suppression because they say it is very safe. It may well be safe to you and me but to someone on an MAOI it can be very dangerous indeed. It is, therefore, important that patients on these drugs realise this, and that the pharmacist issuing such drugs as phenelzine ensures the patient is given instructions not to eat cheese, Bovril, or other tyramine-containing foods or drugs. Tyramine releases noradrenaline from sympathetic nerve endings in patients who are on MAOIs because the tyramine cannot be destroyed by the monoamine oxidase enzyme. Medicines such as nose-drops, inhalations and cold and cough cures containing these sympathomimetic amines are the problems.

We often forget that there is also an interaction of these drugs with narcotic analgesics particularly pethidine. Patients given normal doses of pethidine, if they are on an MAOI, can sustain a very profound central nervous depression. The mechanism is not entirely clear but it is interesting that in experiemental animals in which the synthesis of 5-HT is inhibited by 5-HT receptor blocking drugs this interaction can be reduced or abolished entirely. We know that 5-HT systems are involved with the central action of narcotic drugs and it could be that this interaction involves the fact that there are increased amounts of 5-HT in the brain of patients of MAOIs.

Adverse Reactions of Monoamine Re-Uptake Inhibitors (MARIs)

The mechanism underlying the adverse reactions associated with tricyclic antidepressants or MARIs can be demonstrated by giving an intravenous dose of tyramine to depressed patients treated with amitriptyline and untreated controls and measuring their blood pressure. In the untreated controls the tyramine releases noradrenaline from the sympathetic nerve endings and dose-response curve can be plotted until a 30mm rise in systolic blood pressure has been achieved. In amitriptyline-treated patients, in whom the MARI is blocking the uptake of tyramine, the dose-response curve is shifted to the right.

The important thing to remember is that this effect occurs within a few hours of the first dose of the drug. Furthermore, there is a straight line relationship between tyramine sensitivity and blood level which is apparent within three hours of receiving the first dose of the drug. Dentists and doctors alike need to remind themselves that as soon as a patient is started on one of these drugs all the possible interactions from the re-uptake inhibition follow, and although the patient may take two or three weeks to show any measurable change in their depression, the pharmacological change on uptake is immediate. Perhaps the most important interaction in this context is that between adrenaline and MARIs.

The enhanced pressor response to noradrenaline in patients on tricyclic antidepressants was responsible years ago for several deaths when a local anaesthetic/noradrenaline combination was injected for dental work. Failure to exclude tricyclic antidepressants before administering noradrenaline constitutes negligence today and yet there are still doctors and dentists who give local anaesthetics containing monoamines without first establishing this important contraindication.

The other interaction of importance to remember is that drugs such as imipramine can reverse the effect of some anti-hypertensives such as bethanidine or guanethidine so blood pressure control will be lost in treated patients if they go onto tricyclic antidepressants.

Patients with endogenous depression are organically ill and this is reflected in the abnormal functioning of their autonomic nervous system, especially the noradrenergic system. They respond differently to tyramine injections, and even the platelets of a depressed patient deal with monoamines in a different way from the platelets of a healthy person. The mechanism for this is unclear but one explanation is that it could be due to the different levels of circulating steroids found in depressed patients producing an influence on noradrenergic and cholinergic function.

Whatever the cause, if you take a population of depressed patients they have different blood pressure levels and a different incidence of sudden cardiac deaths and strokes compared with non-depressed populations. So they are different in some way.

Finally, we need to consider the anticholinergic effects of tricyclic antidepressants. Some years ago we measured salivary flow in a group of patients, half of whom were treated with mianserin and the other half with amitriptyline. Amitriptyline initially produced the expected fall in salivation due to its atropine-like action but as we continued treatment and as the patients improved the salivary flow returned to baseline. The interesting thing was that mianserin, which does not actually have an anticholinergic effect, was associated with an increased salivary flow. It was not the mianserin that was producing the increased salivary flow, however, but the fact that patients who are depressed have lower salivation than do non-depressed patients. So it is not just the adrenergic system that is different in depression, but also the cholinergic system. Patients salivate less but as their depression improves so does their salivation. So often in studies that are done this factor is not taken into account. Patients start off at different baselines because their depression is not just in the mind it is very much an organic, physical condition.

The MARIs are thus a very interesting group of drugs with effects on the adrenergic and cholinergic systems together with a membrane stabilising effect on the heart. Whilst this review has not covered all the interactions it behoves us as therapeutists to have some understanding of the mechanisms which underlie unwanted effects and to bear them in mind when evaluating the new drugs that come onto the market.

COGNITIVE AND BEHAVIOURAL CONSEQUENCES OF ANTIDEPRESSANTS

I Hindmarch

Head of Human Psychopharmacology Research Unit, University of Leeds

The effects of antidepressants need not necessarily be of life threatening physiological dimensions to be very disturbing to depressed patients. It is my brief to remind you that it is possible to show differences between antidepressants in the extent to which they disrupt cognitive function and psychological performance and to highlight the clinical relevance of these distinctions.

Unarguably most antidepressants which are currently available are equally efficacious. Choosing between them in a therapeutic situation is, therefore, dependent very much on patient characteristics and on the side effects of the individual drugs. Psychopharmacologists are interested in these drugs because any drug that affects the brain will also disrupt information processing and other psychological functions.

In order to adjust to a psychological environment or solve problems or use mental processes, the brain is constantly integrating "bits" of sensory information and linking them with overt motor responses. Any drug with CNS activity has the potential to interfere with this integrative function, modifying in some way the integrity or the flow of information. It is possible to monitor the effects of antidepressant drugs by observing changes in sensorimotor function. Sensorimotor function, memory and other psychological processes are measured by psychometric tests. These tests have no relevance outside a theoretical model of information processing and although it is impossible to localise information processing in neurological terms, we can deduce patterns of sensory coding and pathways by which information is co-ordinated and integrated into some form of response. Thought processes are, of course, modified by personality, memory, motivation, predisposition and expectations. In conceptualising depressive illness certain theorists (Widlocher, 1983a; 1983b) would see disruption of information processing as a prime manifestation, with affective disturbance as secondary to the cognitive dysfunction.

Over the years tests which measure, in a reliable and consistent way, the effects of drugs on various aspects of information processing have been developed (Hindmarch, 1980). Certain of these are particularly sensitive to the effects of antidepressants and are reliable and replicable for research purposes.

Choice Reaction Time

This is a very simple procedure in which the speed of a simple sensorimotor response is recorded. The patient is asked to press a central button in a console as soon as the stimulus light comes on and to do this as quickly as possible. Variation in speed of response gives a reliable indication of the integrity of the sensorimotor system. By keeping constant the distance the finger has to move from the centre of the console to each of the light stimulus buttons, it is possible to subtract the motor component of the response from the total reaction time indicating the time taken by the patient to process this very simple "bit" of information. Drugs with sedative action will slow down or disturb the rate of information processing and this is manifest by a lengthening of reaction time.

Critical Flicker Fusion Threshold (CFFT)

This is another tried and tested way of measuring rate of information processing. The patient has to observe a flickering light, which is made to flicker faster until it is impossible to distinguish the discrete flashes of light and the patient reports seeing a continuous light. Drugs which disrupt information processing will interfere with the CFF threshold.

The Stroop Effect

This effect relies on the integrity of the interhemispheric transfer of information and is exquisitely sensitive to even the slightest disruption by drugs

The patient is first asked to read a list of colour words - black, green, blue, etc. This is easily accomplished by most people who will then be rendered monosyllabic when they try to name the colours of the ink in which the colour names are printed when the word and the ink colour do not correspond. The task involves ignoring the dominant left hemisphere messages to read the words in favour of the right hemisphere task of naming ink colours.

Tracking Tests

Tracking tests examine the integrity of overt skilled sensorimotor performance. Car handling ability is the ultimate task in this category because it is a real life task which many patients receiving antidepressants are required to perform on a regular basis. Furthermore, in epidemiological studies from Australia, the Netherlands and America, patients on antidepressant drugs are over-represented in fatality statistics. It is an important area for concern and a variety of tests, including high speed car handling tasks and brake reaction time measures in a car driving situation, have been used to assess the effects of drugs in real life.

Subjective Measures

With any of these drugs it is also important to ask the patient how they feel. Such subjective information can be collected by questionnaires or visual analogue scales.

Memory Tests

There are many different tests of memory which are concerned with short-term memory, the so-called executive memory or working memory. It is this aspect of cognitive functioning that gives integrity to all our waking behaviour. Coherence and executive function become impossible if a person is unable to hold a sequence of words in their short-term memory long enough to follow meaning.

It takes little imagination to grasp the impact a disruption in short-term memory might have, particularly in the elderly, who are often the recipients of antidepressant drugs. Short-term memory capacity inevitably deteriorates with age, quite apart from any drug effects, and simple everyday tasks like making telephone calls can become very difficult. If one compounds the problem by administering drugs which further impair mental faculties, normal psychological functioning becomes impossible. Patients may then start to avoid situations where it is necessary to use short-term memory, which only serves to increase their social isolation and feelings of incompetence.

Impaired intellectual functioning is thus not a trivial aspect of antidepressant treatment bearing in mind that depression itself produces primary disturbance in cognitive function and CNS integrity. These effects have considerable implication for the quality of life of the patient who finds their everyday cognitive behaviours disrupted.

The Effects of Antidepressant Drugs on Cognitive Functioning

Table I summarises over 15 years of research into the effects of antidepressant drugs on human performance. I shall select a few representative examples of these studies to discuss in more detail.

The detrimental effects of amitriptyline have been well documented. Clear differences emerged between amitriptyline, zimeldine and placebo-treated subjects tested on the car-braking task (Hindmarch et al., 1983) with much longer reaction times recorded for those on amitriptyline. Amitriptyline also fares badly when the Stroop Test is used to measure performance but not all tricyclics impair performance on this test to the same degree. For example, lofepramine at doses of 70mg and 140mg showed none of the disruptive effects of 50mg of amitriptyline (Hindmarch et al., 1988). There does not seem to be any structure/activity relationship to explain why some tricyclics impair and some do not impair psychometric test performance.

Where memory is concerned the Sternberg test is sensitve enough to pick up the disruptive effects of social doses of alcohol equivalent to one large gin and tonic. Relatively small doses of antidepressants, clinically speaking, can produce effects of similar magnitude when compared with placebo and worse effects when combined with alcohol. We compared 25mg amitriptyline, 10mg mianserin and 50mg trazadone with placebo (Hindmarch and Subhan, 1986). Buproprion, interestingly, has absolutely no effect at all on this memory test.

Table I

	mg	CFF	CRT	STM IPR	SUB SED	SIM CAR	OTR CAR	ALC
Amitriptyline	50	●	●	●	●	●	●	●
Mianserin	10	●	●	●	●	●	●	●
Trazodone	50	●	●	●	●	●	●	●
Dothiepin	50	◐	◐	◐	●	◐		●
Desipramine	50	◐	◐	◐	●	◐		
Lofepramine	140	◐	◐		◐	◐		
Zimeldine	200	◐	◐	◐	◐	◐	◐	
Midalcipran	100	◐	◐	◐	◐	◐		◐
Buproprion	100	◐	◐		◐	◐	◐	○
Fluoxetine	40	○	◐	◐	◐	◐		
Sertraline	100	○	◐	◐	◐	◐		
Paroxetine	30	○	◐	◐	◐	◐		●?
Nomifensine	100	○		○	○	○	◐	

Legend

● = significant impairment on these functions when compared to placebo controls
◐ = no significant difference between the treatment and placebo
○ = significant improvement on these measures compared to placebo treatments
? = limited information and/or ambiguous data
CFF = Critical Flicker Fusion Threshold
CRT = Choice Reaction Time
STM IPR = Short Term Memory Information Processing
SUB SED = Subjective Ratings of Sedation
SIM CAR = Simulated Car Driving
OTR CAR = On-the-road Car Driving
ALC = Evidence that the effects are potentiated by doses of alcohol (0.5g/kg body weight)

Similar results were recorded in a tracking task where the same drugs were compared and, once again, buproprion showed none of the detrimental effects of the other substances. It is noteworthy that the detrimental effects are seen across a wide spectrum of skills, they are not confined to a single test. 50mg amitriptyline, for example, will significantly impair tracking, reaction time, brake reaction time, increase drowsiness and impair CFF threshold (Hindmarch et al., 1983).

Critical flicker fusion has actually proven to be a very sensitive and interesting measure - so sensitive, in fact, that it can detect differences between imipramine n-oxide, amitriptyline n-oxide and amitriptyline over a period of hours (Hindmarch, 1982). CFF can also differentiate quite clearly between nomifensine, placebo and amitriptyline. Amitriptyline produces a significant decrement in CFF and nomifensine has absolutely no effect at all (Hindmarch, 1988).

In order to differentiate between anticholinergic side effects and simple sedation mianserin (no anticholinergic activity), amitriptyline and desiprimine (anticholinergic) and nomifensine (also no anticholinergic activity) were compared against placebo. Using CFF thresholds as an index of impairment it was obvious that both amitriptyline and mianserin caused significant problems with information processing. We deduced, therefore, that much of the observed disruption could be attributed to the effects of sedation, as desipramine, a tricyclic drug, had no detrimental effect of CFFT. This phenomenon is seen not only in the laboratory but can also be replicated in patient populations. Kahn et al. (1985) recorded CFF thresholds in hospitalised patients being treated with either nomifensine or mianserin and his results were identical to those found in laboratory studies. Hanks (1985) looked at CFF scores over a seven week treatment period with amitriptyline. The decrement in performance was not only significant but prolonged. This is a very important aspect to remember because unlike tolerance to the anticholinergic side effects of amitriptyline e.g. dry mouth etc., which gradually develops, a patient's cognitive functions are impaired for the duration of treatment. A patient's mental competence and psychological ability to help themselves is reduced by the treatment designed to help them, this has important implications for the treatment of depressed patients.

Conclusion

The implications are quite staightforward as far as the effects of antidepressant drugs on cognitive functioning are concerned. It would seem to be good medicine, assuming that the various antidepressants available are clinically equipotent, to use drugs from the summary table (Table I) which are the least disruptive for the patient. You can see a quite clear three-fold division - some substances incontrovertibly impair psychological performance, car driving and cognitive functions, some substances do not and a few appear to augment performance. Since antidepressants are to be prescribed to ambulant outpatients only drugs with no effects on these important measures of patient behaviour should be considered.

References

1. Hanks, G.W. (1985) The effects of amitriptyline and nomifensine on critical flicker fusion threshold in an elderly patient population. The Royal Society of Medicine International Congress and Symposium Series No. 70, 95 - 97.
2. Hindmarch, I. (1980) Psychomotor function and psychoactive drugs. British Journal of Clinical Pharmacology, 10, 145 - 150.
3. Hindmarch, I. (1982) Antidepressant drugs and performance. British Journal of Clinical Practice, Suppl. 19, 73 - 77.
4. Hindmarch, I., Subhan, Z. and Stoker, M.J. (1983) The effects of zimeldine and amitriptyline on car driving and psychomotor performance. Acta Psychiatrica Scandinavica, Suppl. 308, 68, 141 - 146.
5. Hinmarch, I. (1986) The effects of psychoactive drugs on car handling and related psychomotor ability: A review. In O'Hanlon, J.F. and de Gier, J.J. (Eds.) Drugs and Driving, pp 71 - 82. Taylor and Francis: London.
6. Hindmarch, I. and Subhan, Z. (1986) The effects of antidepressants, taken in conjunction with alcohol, on information processing and psychomotor performance related to car driving ability. In O'Hanlon, J.F. and de Gier, J.J. (Eds.) Drugs and Driving, pp 231 - 240. Taylor and Francis: London
7. Hindmarch, I., Harrison, C. and Shillingford, C.A. (1988) An investigation of the effects of lofepramine, nomifensine, amitriptyline and placebo on aspects of memory and psychomotor performance related to car driving. International Clinical Psychopharmacology (In Press)
8. Khan, M.C., Mahapatra, S.N., Stonier, P.D. and Thomas, E.M. (1985) Nomifensine and mianserin: non-tricyclic antidepressants with distinct clinical profiles: a randomised double-blind study. The Royal Society of Medicine International Congress and Symposium Series No. 70, 71 - 76.
9. Widlocher, D. (1983a) Psychomotor retardation: clinical, theoretical and psychometric aspects. Psychiatric Clinics of North America, 6, (1), 27 - 39.
10. Widlocher, D. (1983b) La ralentissement depressif. Presses Universitaires de France: Paris

Discussion

Turner: With regard to the augmenting effect of nomifensine, we too have recorded similar results, not only with nomifensine, but also with cyclazindol and mazindol, which are marketed as anti-obesity drugs. The subjective experience after taking any of these compounds is of an amphetamine-like action. Do you share my concern that these compounds are potential drugs of abuse?

Hindmarch: What you say is interesting but there has been no evidence from animal studies to show that dependency developed when nomifensine was added to their food. It did not have the same addictive potential as amphetamine at all. In our human studies the augmentation seen with nomifensine was far less than that seen with amphetamine and I have never seen fit to describe nomifensine as a "stimulant" drug. It is "mentalerting" in the same way as a strong cup of coffee.

Turner: We have recently reviewed all our research data as you have done and found that visual analogue scales produced just as consistent and reproducible results as other tests. Is it, therefore, necessary to use such sophisticated tests as yours to show these effects?

Hindmarch: I could not agree with you more about visual analogue scales provided thay are properly designed. However, there is no reason why CFF thresholds should not be more widely used. Very simple machines are now commercially available which provide good, objective, psychometric data for clinical trials. Visual analogues, I agree, make a good adjunctive response measure.

Audience: Could you comment on the time course of sedation on cognitive performance. There is some evidence that with drugs like amitriptyline the cognitive inhibition continues over weeks, whereas, say with mianserin after 7 days it wears off, which implies that sedation may not be the real trigger.

Hindmarch: I would agree with you. Hanks has shown the effects of amitriptyline persisting for 7 weeks. In the Kahn study on mianserin the CFF deficit was lessening at the end of a week's treatment. It does seem that there is something else as well as sedation. Certainly with our work on benzodiazepines we have shown that it is possible to have sedative benzodiazepines which are amnestic and to have non-sedative benzodiazepines which are also amnestic, so whatever is disrupting short-term information processing, it is not just sedation.

Henry: I was interested to see that your volunteers on placebo improved as the day went on. Is this a circadian effect or attributable to a learning effect during the course of the day?

Hindmarch: You can get both things. A lot depends on the particular population of volunteers. One of my students recently wrote a PhD thesis on the effects of circadian rhythms on CFFT. It is sensitive enough to pick up circadian rhythms especially the early afternoon dip. You do need larger populations for demonstrating circadian effects than those used normally in cross-over drug studies. We can, however, exclude learning effects from all of our studies. Firstly, the volunteers are trained before entering the studies and, secondly, the CFFT test equipment and technique seems to be free from practice effects.

ANTIDEPRESSANTS AND THE ELDERLY

P Crome

Consultant Physician in Geriatric Medicine
Orpington Hospital

and

Clinical Associate Professor
Department of Medicine, University of Saskatchewan

Why discuss the elderly? Firstly, the elderly comprise a large section of the population and the numbers are increasing, especially of those aged over 75 and over 85. The numbers are expected to level out but not for another 50 years or so. Secondly, depression in old age is common. Depending on how you define it, between 10 - 60% of the elderly population may be suffering from one sort of depression or another. Thirdly, there are special aetiological factors such as social isolation, bereavement, poor physical health and poverty, all of which are common in old age. Fourthly, and the subject of this paper, there are problems with medication.

Some of the earliest papers on imipramine presaged things to come. "Blood pressure is scarcely affected by imipramine. If, however, there is arterial hypertension then in many cases imipramine lowers it slightly. We have seen differences of up to 70 mmHg" (Kuhn, 1958). If that is "slight" I wonder what he would have considered to be "moderate" let alone "severe". He then goes on, "we observed collapse phenomena only very occasionally"! Lehmann et al's (1958) paper of the same year in the Canadian Psychiatric Association Journal reported side effects in one third of all patients but in more than half of those aged 65 and over. Side effects reported included syncope and hypotension, epilepsy, other neurological abnormalities including diplopia, jerky tremors and involuntary staring. Psychiatric complications included hallucinations. Anticholinergic effects were also reported. Thus, in these two early papers, not only had most of the side effects of the drugs been identified, but also the elderly had been noted to be more susceptible.

Cardiovascular Side-Effects of Antidepressants
1. Postural Hypotension

Muller et al in 1961 compared the cardiovascular effects of imipramine in patients aged 60 and over who had a variety of cardiovascular diseases with patients aged below 60 without significant cardiovascular problems (Table I).

Table I Effects of Imipramine on Standing Blood Pressure

Age	No.	No Change	↓	↑	Hypotention Slight	Mod	Severe	Withdrawn
> 60 yrs	41	9	32	0	15	7	10	10
< 60 yrs	41	24	15	2	12	3	0	0

Of the 41 patients over 60 years, three-quarters experienced a drop in blood pressure. The "slight" decrease group (5 - 20 mmHg drop) was not associated with symptoms but those with "moderate" decrease (10 - 20 mmHg) experienced dizziness, weakness, sweating and fainting. In the ten patients with "severe" falls in blood pressure (20 - 80 mmHg, average 40 mmHg) symptoms included moderate shock and prolonged, severe weakness necessitating discontinuation of the drug. Below 60 years the pattern of response was quite different. Recumbent blood pressure remained unaltered in both groups. The concern over hypotension in old people is not just about unpleasant symptoms such as fainting but also about the likelihood of injuries sustained whilst falling, particularly wrist and femoral neck fractures, and even more seriously, of strokes resulting from decreased cerebral blood perfusion.

The impaired blood pressure response to changes in posture in the elderly is exacerbated by drugs. Neshkes et al (1985) found doxepin differed little from placebo in this respect but imipramine showed a marked effect (Table II).

Table II
Postural Hypotension Before and After Antidepressants

Orthostatic Drop	Imipramine	Doxepin	Placebo
1. Before treatment	13.2/3	16.4/5.9	16.9/5.0
2. After treatment	25.9/7.3	10.5/1.2	12.4/2.0

Christensen et al (1985) showed that patients do eventually become tolerant to postural hypotension. Elderly depressed patients treated with amitriptyline experienced initial orthostatic hypotension which then decreased in amplitude and duration over four weeks.

2. Myocardial Effects

In the previously mentioned study by Muller et al (1961), there were four patients who developed cardiac failure and two who had myocardial infarctions. There have also been many single case reports of cardiac decompensation in patients with pre-existing cardiovascular disease whilst they have been on tricyclic antidepressants. In view of their known experimental effects on heart muscle it is reasonable to assume that there is some reduction in myocardial function. This may be compensated by tachycardia. Whether this problem is any worse in the elderly than in younger individuals is not clear.

3. Arrhythmias
Tricyclic antidepressants are known to cause electrocardiographic changes. In Christensen's study in the elderly the PQ, QRS and corrected QT intervals were all significantly prolonged at 4 weeks. Unlike the changes in blood pressure, this effect persisted over the four weeks of the study. There have been numerous other studies detailing individual cases of arrhythmias with most of the tricyclic antidepressants now available. The influence of age as opposed to pre-existing cardiac disease is not known.

4. Sudden Death
In the early 1970's the Aberdeen Group (Coull et al, 1970; Moir et al, 1972) reported that cardiac patients receiving amitriptyline had an increased rate of sudden death. 13 out of 119 amitriptyline treated patients, compared with only 3 in a control group, died suddenly. Subsequently the Boston Collaborative Drug Surveillance Program (1972) failed to substantiate these findings and the majority view now favours the Boston conclusion rather than the Aberdeen one. Personally, I tend to use the non-tricyclic antidepressants in patients with active cardiac disease but I do not regard controlled cardiac disease in the elderly to be an absolute contraindication to tricyclic antidepressant use.

Table III
Other Side-Effects of Antidepressants

* Sedation
* Fatigue
* Confusion
* Dry mouth
* Retention of urine
* Constipation
  Paralysis of accomodation
* Raised intra-occular pressure
* Tremor
  Weight gain

(* occur more frequently in the elderly)

The clinical significance of this increased incidence of side effects is clear e.g. prostatic hypertrophy is a disease of the old and not the young. Constipation is common in the elderly. Glaucoma is also a disease of old age.

Causes of Side Effects in the Elderly
Drug side effects may be due to a number of factors:-
1. Impairment of homeostatic mechanisms (N.B. in relation to postural hypotension).
2. Drug interactions. Elderly people are the major recipients of most of the common classes of drugs.

3. Alterations in pharmacokinetics.
4. Alterations in drug sensitivity i.e. the effects of the same amount of drug at a receptor, cell and whole organ level differ in the elderly. This has been shown for benzodiazepines and for warfarin but not for antidepressants.
5. Non-compliance. With the elderly it is much more likely that patients will take too few tablets rather than too many.

Side effects would, in fact, be such more common if patients took their medication correctly. Prescribing drugs once a day, and most antidepressants can be prescribed once a day, improves compliance dramatically. A community study of the elderly in the North Southwark area found that 94% of drugs prescribed once a day, in the morning, were taken correctly; 71% of drugs taken once daily in the evening were taken correctly, but when one came to drugs to be taken three times a day only 25% were taken correctly. We also know that many patients have misconceptions about their medication and that time talking to the patient about their drugs, their purpose, when and how they should be taken and what to do if there are side effects, is time well spent.

Pharmacokinetics of Antidepressants in the Elderly

The ageing body undergoes many physiological changes which potentially, at least, can effect the way in which drugs are handled. There is a reduction in gastric acid production, gastro-intestinal motility, gastro-intestinal blood flow and absorptive surfaces, all of which may affect drug absorption. There is an increase in the proportion of the body which is fat and a decrease in body water. Plasma albumin, to which many drugs are bound, is reduced, and alpha-1-acid-glycoprotein which binds some antidepressants is increased. Metabolism of drugs may be affected by liver size, liver blood and hepatic metabolic capacity. Finally, excretion in the kidneys may be reduced by reductions in glomerular filtration and renal tubular function. In addition to these physiological changes, pathological changes in the gastro-intestinal tract, the cardiovascular system, the liver and the kidneys may all also affect drug handling.

Pharmacokinetic studies of young and elderly subjects show that, as a general rule, the half-life of tricyclic antidepressants is prolonged and the clearance is reduced. The significance of a prolonged half-life is that it will take longer for the drug to reach steady-state and possibly longer for any side effects to wear off. A drug has to be given for approxiamtely four to five half-lives before steady-state is reached so that, for some of these drugs, this means a couple of weeks or so, as in the case of desipramine. Clearance is the sole physiological determinant of steady-state plasma concentration. Thus, if the clearance is lower, then the steady-state level will be higher, and this has been the finding for amitriptyline, nortriptyline, imipramine and desipramine. Superimposed on this general reduction in metabolism is a much greater variation between elderly people in their response to antidepressants.

Metabolism may also be impaired by the co-administration of other drugs which are likely to be given to elderly people such as propranolol, which inhibits the metabolism of maprotiline, presumably by lowering cardiac output and thus the rate of delivery of drug to the liver. The enzymes responsible for metabolising these drugs may be impaired by other drugs. Major tranquillisers, for example, have been shown to cause higher imipramine, desipramine and nortriptyline steady-state concentrations. Thus it is, that the elderly who are given antidepressants, are quite likely to be already taking other drugs which affect the metabolism of tricyclic compounds.

Tricyclic antidepressants undergo extensive first-pass metabolism. In the elderly this tends to be impaired which results in higher plasma drug concentrations and may, in turn, explain why side effects may be greater when the drug is first given. Tricyclic antidepressants are frequently degraded to metabolites which are themselves active such as nortriptyline from amitriptyline and desipramine from imipramine. In general these metabolites have longer half-lives than their parent compounds. It therefore takes longer for the metabolites as well as the parent compounds to reach steady-state. The same holds true for the hydroxymetabolites, concentrations of which have been shown to be higher in elderly people. This probably occurs because the hyroxymetabolites are excreted by the kidney whose capacity to do so is reduced even in elderly people without obvious renal disease.

In summary the changes likely to be seen are:-

1. increased variability
2. reduced rate of hepatic biotransformation
3. prolongation of plasma half-life
4. higher steady-state levels on repeated dosing
5. reduced first-past metabolism

New Antidepressants in the Elderly

1. Fluvoxamine

A single dose study (Duphar, 1984) showed no difference in maximum recorded plasma concentration, area under the plasma concentration time curve, half-life or clearance between a group of young and elderly subjects. A multiple dose study (Duphar, 1985a) showed that there was no difference in pre-dose concentrations on days 5, 10, 14 and 28 of multiple dosing indicating that steady-state was reached within 5 days and there were no differences between these values and those for younger subjects subjected to a similar protocol. A retrospective analysis of patients in clinical trials (Duphar, 1985b) showed that steady-state plasma concentrations in patients aged over 60 were similar to those in patients aged 60 at dose ranges of 100 to 300 mg a day.

2. Mianserin

With mianserin, Shami et al (1983) found that the terminal elimination half-life was prolonged and the apparent oral clearance was reduced.

The differences were quite large and again the variability was greater in the elderly. Similar conclusions were reported by Altamura et al (1982). One negative study by Maguire et al (1983) showed that the half-life was increased by 50% but this did not reach statistical significance.

3. Trazodone

Again elimination half-life, area under the plasma concentration time curve and clearance were all altered. Miller et al (1987) studied men and women separately and found that these measurements were altered in men and not in women. Generally similarly impaired metabolism has been shown for viloxazine.

Conclusions

The elderly are at greater risk of side effects from antidepressants as they are from many other drugs. We know that the pharmacokinetics are altered in old age. This is probably the major factor in drug toxicity. On a practical level I would suggest that doses at least half, if not a third, of standard are prescribed for all those aged 75 and over. Finally, of course, it is important to remember that one treats individual people and not groups and that the specifics of treatment, the drug, the dose, the duration of treatment must be considered on an individual basis.

References

1. Altamura A., Melerio T., Invernizzi G. and Gomeni R. (1982). Influence of age on mianserin pharmacokinetics. Psychopharmacology 78: 380 - 382.
2. Boston Collaborative Drug Surveillance Program. (1972). Adverse reactions to the tricyclic-antidepressant drugs. Lancet i: 529 - 531.
3. Christensen P., Thomsen H.Y., Pedersen O.L., Thayssen P., Oxhoej H., Kragh-Sorensen P. and Gram L.F. (1985). Cardiovascular effects of amitriptyline in the treatment of elderly depressed patients. Psychopharmacology 87: 212 - 215.
4. Coull D.C., Crooks J., Dingwall-Fordyce I., Scott A.M. and Weir R.D. (1970). Amitriptyline and cardiac disease. Lancet ii: 590 - 591.
5. Duphar Report No H. 114.621 (1984). Duphar, Weesp.
6. Duphar Report No H. 114.622 (1985a). Duphar, Weesp.
7. Duphar Report No H. 114.623 (1985b). Duphar, Weesp.
8. Kuhn R. (1958). The treatment of depressive states with G 22355 (imipramine hydrochloride). American Journal of Psychiatry 115: 459 - 464.
9. Lehmann H.E., Cahn C.H. and de Verteuil R.L. (1958). The treatment of depressive conditions with imipramine (G 22355). Canadian Psychiatric Association Journal 3: 155 - 164.
10. Maguire K.M., McIntyre I., Nporman T. and Burrows G.D. (1983). The pharmacokinetics of mianserin in elderly depressed patients. Psychiatry Research 8: 281 - 287.
11. Miller L.G., Greenblatt D.J., Friedman H., Burstein E., Scavone J.M., Harmatz, J.S. and Shader R.I. (1987). Trazodone kinetics in old age. Clinical Pharmacology and Therapeutics 41: 210.
12. Moir, D.C., Cornwell W.B., Dingwall-Fordyce I., Crooks J., O'Malley K., Turnbull M.J. and Weir R.D. (1972). Cardiotoxicity of amitriptyline. Lancet ii: 561 - 564.
13. Muller O.F., Goodman N. and Bellet S. (1961). The hypotensive effect of imipramine hydrochloride in patients with cardiovascular disease. Clinical Pharmacology and Therapeutics 2: 300 - 307.

14. Neshkes R., Gerner R., Jarvik L., Mintz J., Joseph J., Linde S., Aldrich J., Conolly M., Rosen R. and Hill M. (1985). Orthostatic effect of imipramine and doxepin in depressed geriatric outpatients. Journal of Clinical Psychopharmacology 5: 102 - 106.
15. Shami M., Elliott H.L., Kelman A.W. and Whiting B. (1983). The pharmacokinetics of mianserin. British Journal of Clinical Pharmacology 30: 239 . 242.

DISCUSSION

Bridges: I am particularly enthusiastic about using clomipramine in high doses for treating cases of resistant depression. Clomipramine differs from other antidepressants in the dose-dependence of its effects. Does this dose-dependency have any pharmacological significance that might be clinically relevant.

Leonard: There are a number of problems in interpreting the overdose figures for clomipramine, not least being the different clinical profiles of patients usually prescribed this drug. It tends to be reserved for the treatment of atypical depressions which means it is less likely to be consumed in overdoses in quite the same way as other tricyclics. From the pharmacological point of view it is a serotonin uptake inhibitor and its major metabolite probably also blocks noradrenaline re-uptake which may or may not be relevant. It also has a quinidine-like membrane stabilising action but whether this differs in potency from the other tricyclics is unknown. To me it remains something of a pharmacological mystery.

Henry: There is not much difference in membrane stabilising activity between clomipramine and the other tricyclics. There is, however, a much more pronounced interaction between clomipramine and the MAOIs than with other tricyclics. We are currently reporting a case of a patient who was taking amitriptyline and tranylcypromine and mistakenly had one tablet of clomipramine substituted for his amitriptyline. The result was a massive, acute reaction, so clomipramine obviously has a very different pharmacological profile. Why its toxicological profile should be so different in terms of mortality statistics I do not know.

Bridges: As the dose increases what happens to the half-life? I find it varies considerably.

Leonard: Obviously, there are changes in half-life associated with ageing which, no doubt, reflects differences in metabolism and excretion which are not directly related to dose. Much of the work on drug half-lives is done in healthy young volunteers and there are dangers in extrapolating from such artificial data to the clinical situation in which sick people take drugs for long periods of time.

Audience: Has Dr Bridges ever used intravenous clomipramine, for example, in patients who refuse E.C.T. or who are sensitive to other antidepressants?

Bridges: As far as I know there is no advantage to intravenous administration of tricyclics as there are no problems with absorption or distribution.

Turner: I can see no advantage other than for psychological reasons. Do you have any experience with intravenous administration?

Bridges: No, I cannot see any indication but it certainly used to be given in this way as a form of treatment.

Turner: Perhaps with intravenous administration there would be a less rapid use of first pass active metabolites and an augmented initial effect on the 5HT system. Is that possible?

Leonard: It is possible but very speculative. There is no indication for this form of therapy unless, perhaps, patients with atypical kinds of depression respond better to the psychological aspects of intravenous drugs.

Audience: Controlled trials have shown no difference in onset of action, potency or efficacy for intravenous versus oral administration of trycyclics either within or between drugs.

Bridges: Its a practise which has largely died out now.

Audience: In this country perhaps, but it is still quite common in France, Italy, Spain and southern mediterranean countries.

Turner: J P Griffin, analysing the number of lines on prescriptions presented by the elderly, concluded that ADRs are not increased in the elderly. He felt that elderly people are not more susceptible to drugs in terms of adverse reactions but that problems arise as a result of polypharmacy. Does Peter Crome go along with that?

Crome: In principle yes, but number of prescriptions *per se* is only part of the equation, it does not take dosage into account or the rationality of prescribing habits. At least doctors are now becoming aware of the special precautions necessary to prescibe safely for the elderly. I wonder how many of our present audience actually prescribe antidepressants differently in the elderly?

Audience: Is there any likelihood that a patient suffering side effects from the tricyclics could bring a malpractise suit against a doctor for not prescribing one of the safer more modern antidepressants?

Crome: I still use the ordinary tricyclic antidepressants and I firmly believe that if they are used sensibly you will not run into problems.

Bridges: There is a danger here that the safest drug may not necessarily be the most potent. By using a more potent drug, albeit, with more side effects to bring depression more rapidly under control you may prevent a suicide.

Ashford: What do you mean "more potent"? To my knowledge there has actually been no difference in efficacy between the antidepressant drugs developed over the past 30 years.

Leonard: Physicians and psychiatrists often say that they use amitriptyline because it is clearly the most potent antidepressant available. But in terms of objectively measured potency from properly controlled clinical trials in hospital and general practise settings, there is no real difference between the drugs. As a pharmacologist I have to say there is no objective evidence that any drug is superior in terms of potency to amitriptyline.

That being the case, one has to do a cost benefit analysis in deciding whether to leave a patient untreated and at risk of suicide, or to treat them and make the best of the side effects. Non-compliance is a major factor in general practise where most of these drugs are prescribed, and this is worse with the tricyclics where the side effects are not well tolerated, particularly in the elderly. By and large I would still favour using the newer antidepressants.

Audience: How long should one continue prescribing antidepressants - 6 months, 9 months, 1 or 2 years?

Bridges: There is no hard data about this but from my own experience there are two points to bear in mind. Firstly, as a clinical consideration I would treat patients longer depending on the severity of their original illness. Secondly, I am very aware that in managing depression we are not curing a disease but easing symptoms during an illness that will spontaneously remit within 6 months to 2 - 2.5 years.

Crome: Likewise, with the elderly, there is no factual information to guide us. Some elderly people may, in fact, suffer prolonged periods of depression which may never spontaneously remit. Whether antidepressants are useful for this group I do not know. In practical terms I would keep patients who have responded to an antidepressant on treatment for 6 months then try and withdraw the drug.

Leonard: Coppen and his group did a nice study involving a double-blind crossover design in which low dose lithium was used after 6 months treatment with a conventional antidepressant. They reported low dose lithium, which has minimal side effects, was found to be particularly beneficial in preventing relapse.

Audience: Several long-term controlled studies which I have seen for periods of 6 months, 1 and 2 years, have shown tricyclics or lithium to be bether than placebo in preventing relapse.

Audience: Is there any evidence that these drugs lose their potency if used for longer than 6 months?

Bridges: Not in my experience. If a patient relapses I increase the dose. With very severe, refractory illnessess, once they are under control they remain so for quite long periods of time.

Turner: There is no pharmacological reason to expect changes. Postsynaptic and presynaptic monoamine receptor density changes 3 - 4 weeks after initiating treatment, and then remains at these levels.

Leonard: Yes, as long as the drug is present this neurotransmitter adaptation persists and it correlates well with the clinical effects of the drug. The adaptation persists after the drug is withdrawn provided the patient remains well, but as soon as they become depressed again biochemical changes in receptors can be measured.

Hindmarch: In this context it is salutory to remember that there are problems inherent in the very way we measure changes over time. Even with a rating scale as good as the Hamilton-D, there are biases inherent in the measuring tool itself where repeated judgements are ellicited over long periods of time. Rating scales are crude instruments - they are not very sensitive to change over time - and what might appear to be loss of efficacy of a drug over time may be more a function of the complexity of the rating instrument.

Turner: I would like to re-emphasise a point I made earlier that depressed patients are organically ill. It has been suggested that some of the results attributed to drugs are really epiphenomena of the underlying disease states. A depressed person, for example, may have had sleep disturbance, appetite changes, body weight changes, altered steroid secretion and disturbed sex hormone production and cycles for many months. All these will interact with treatment. As they improve you would expect their weight, sleep and endocrine system to return towards normality. Dosage may need adjustment in response to these physical changes.

Audience: Tricyclics with few toxic side effects, such as dothiepin, seem to be more dangerous in overdose than clomipramine which has many side effects. Why should this be?

Leonard: This anomaly has also been of concern to me. Objectively, dothiepin would seem to be the safer drug and yet it has such a bad record for overdosage. John Henry's work on the membrane stabilising action of dothiepin and its effect in causing sudden heart block may account for its toxicity in overdose.

Audience: Professor Leonard's league table type of analysis of drug toxicity in overdose appears to be somewhat simplistic to me. If people fail to kill themselves with one of the newer, reputedly safer antidepressants, a certain proportion of them may still manage to kill themselves by switching to an alternative method.

Leonard: Suicidal ideation is an integral part of severe depression and, therefore, it concerns us all as clinicians and pharmacologists that we do not encourage a patient to exercise their right to kill themselves by taking an overdose of the drugs designed to treat them. Simplistic as my analysis may be, it utilises the only facts available to us.

Audience: It is very difficult to get a coherent picture when all you have to go on is the mortality statistics themselves with no additional clinical or psychological details. Remarkably similar results for the toxicity of antidepressants were obtained using a completely different data-base such as John Henry's prescription data analysis.

Audience: Does the panel recommend giving tricyclics three times a day or as a single dose at night?

Crome: With regard to the elderly patient the single nocturnal dose creates problems such as quite severe postural hypotension when the old person gets up to void.

Hindmarch: There are also well documented effects of antidepressants on patterns of sleep. REM sleep is reduced by antidepressant so that as the drug effects decrease REM urgency occurs and there is evidence now to show that this can be associated with respiratory distress. Before giving patients their drugs as a single nocturnal dose we need to know much more about these serious apnoeic and respiratory effects.

Bridges: Physicians and psychiatrists, in general, seem to try and avoid using lithium with elderly people, whereas many psychogeriatricians say they experience no difficulties at all with using it. What is Dr Crome's experience with lithium in the elderly?

Crome: Since 10% of the elderly are on diuretics I think it is quite hazardous to use lithium in this combination. It is perhaps safe if frequently monitored but I would not use it for patients with concomitant physical disease.

Audience: How far should we warn patients on tricyclic antidepressants not to drive? London Transport do not allow anyone to drive who is taking psychotropic drug which has important implications for long-term maintenance therapy.

Hindmarch: If you were in court defending your clinical judgement over a medico-legal issue involving amitriptyline I would be acting for the prosecution. If you had prescribed one of the newer drugs I would be on your side.

Audience: So far there has not been such a case.

Hindmarch: No, but in America there have been successful prosecutions where benzodiazepines have been involved and the material I have presented today clearly shows the detrimental effects of some antidepressants on car handling performance. The recommendations of the civil aviation authorities provide a useful guide for clinical practise. These list the drugs which are not compatible with flying and the period of time for which the pilot is grounded if he has taken them. All antidepressants will effect cognitive functioning to some extend so, in the clinical situation, all you can do is select the most effective drug with the least disruptive activity and try and match the drug profile to the individual patient's needs.

Audience: The Chief Medical Officer at London Transport said he would view sympathetically the use of lithium.

Hindmarch: When talking about the effects of drugs on driving let us not forget their role in fatal accidents. Epidemiological studies from Australia and New Zealand implicate antidepressant drugs in 35% of all motor vehicle accidents involving fatalities. The data is very "soft" but even if we assume that only 10% of accidents are associated with antidepressants this is still horrendous. It is only the tip of the iceberg in terms of "behavioural toxicity". It ignores the whole range of fatal domestic accidents, accidents involving pedestrians and industrial accidents which we have no way of taking into account. The true picture of toxicity of each drug is far more complex than we can objectively show but this soft data is indicating important differences between drugs which we should heed.

Dawling: At the Poisons Unit we are currently doing a study with the Department of Transport of the association between tricyclics and fatal accidents and are finding a very much lower incidence - around 0.05%.

Hindmarch: This is fascinating - are your results published yet?

Dawling: No, the study is not yet complete.

Hindmarch: The difference in statistics is amazing. Why they should be so low in the U.K. when the New Zealand study was around 30% and studies in Scandinavia have produced figure of 10 - 12% I do not know, unless it reflects a difference in sampling procedures.

Audience: Benzodiazepine were involved in 1% of fatal accidents and ethanol in 25 - 30%. Perhaps the difference is between fatal accidents and all accidents, but I think we would run into ethical problems of sampling them.

Hindmarch: You are right but it would provide us with very valuable information if it could be done.

FAILURE TO TREAT DEPRESSION

A W Clare

Professor and Head of Department of Psychological Medicine
St Bartholomew's Hospital, London

Our major research interest at St. Bartholomew's Hospital has been depression, but more particularly, depression in the primary care setting, the reason for this being that by far the greatest proportion of affective disorder, however defined, presents to the GP. Only a small proportion, usually at the more severe end of the spectrum, comes to psychiatrists and presents in the hospital setting.

Nevertheless, ten or more years of research into depression in the primary care setting has not gone much beyond clarifying some of the epidemiology of psychiatric morbidity in primary care. We know, for example, that around 15% of presentations are for this problem and that there are two main groups of patients: those with acute, short-lived disturbances and those with more chronic conditions. How many of the first group go on to become the second is still unknown. We also know that the majority of people with depression are dealt with in general practice, that they present with such elusive diagnostic profiles that they are often classified by psychiatrists as mixed anxiety-depressive states (which is little more than a descriptive diagnosis) and that attempts to classify depression in primary care more appropriately continue.

Our own research has been designed to look at several questions:-

1. Using standard psychiatric diagnostic criteria such as DSM III, what proportion of the psychiatric morbidity in primary care would be designated as severe or major depressive illness?
2. What proportion of the totality of depressed patients fall into this category?
3. What is the natural history and outcome of primary care depression?
4. What role does treatment play?

Severity of Depression

There has been a tendency in the past to look on depression in primary care as a somewhat mild and transitory phenomenon - a view that was supported by the findings of Sireling et al (1985) in their study comparing depressed patients in general practice with their counterparts attending psychiatric outpatient clinics. Not only did the general practice depressive appear to be less severely ill but they also had shorter episodes of depression and there was a lower incidence of primary and endogenous depression.

Whilst these conclusions are inescapable from the data they present, they give a less than complete picture of the situation as it actually exists in general practice. The study suffers from one of the problems inherent in all attempts to characterise depression in primary care and that is one of sampling bias. For example, all patients already taking antidepressants were excluded from the study as were all those who had recently received a psychiatric opinion. Furthermore, one fifth of the patients in the general practice group either had no depressive symptoms at all or were actually suffering from other disorders. So the sample can hardly be considered to be fully representative, which is a great pity because its conclusions continue to give credence to the belief that depression in primary care tends to be mild and self-limiting.

Brown et al (1985) controlled for a number of these factors and found considerable overlap between the severity of depressive disorders in psychiatric outpatients and in the community. What distinguished the two, it seems, was not the severity of disorder but the way the symptoms were expressed. GPs tend to make decisions about referral of depressed patients not so much on the basis of the severity of illness but on the presence of additional complicating factors such as personality difficulties, alcohol abuse, failure to respond to treatment or threats of self-harm.

Our own contribution to the study of the nature and prevalence of severe depressive disorder in general practice involved an intensive study of over 2,000 consultations in a North London Health Centre using the General Health Questionnaire, the SADS and the PSE and applying a variety of diagnostic criteria. A profile of diagnoses has been generated and it is clear that around 5% of consecutive attenders in the setting of general practice are easily classified as suffering from major depressive disorder. In addition, a further 4 - 5% can be classified as a milder form of depressive disorder. These figures resemble the percentages reported in a number of United States studies and confirm that, indeed, a considerable proportion, 1 in 20, of patients presenting to general practitioners are manifesting clearcut depressive illness of a significant nature.

Research in General Practice

Given the extent of the problem the next issue concerns what we should be doing about major depressive illness. GPs want to know whether they should be treating it, and if so, should they be using antidepressants with all their disadvantages and what is the evidence that this does any good anyway? These reasonable questions are not that easy to answer - the problems involved in undertaking antidepressant studies in the real world of general practice, as distinct from the controlled world of the hospital clinical trial have proven formidable indeed.

For example, we looked to see how many of the 196 depressed patients we identified in primary care would meet the inclusion criteria for a classical antidepressant drug trial. After eliminating the too young and the elderly, those suffering from other psychiatric disorders, alcohol abuse, co-existing physical diseases, the pregnant and those who would not consent we ended up with 22 patients - not a very representative sample but typical of what would be studied in a classical controlled trial. Nevertheless, a number of studies do suggest that the appropriate use of antidepressants in treatment of depression in general practice is a therapeutically effective intervention.

What are the consequences of failure to treat major depressive illness? To answer that one needs good natural history studies of psychiatric morbidity in general practice which, until recently, have been rather lacking. Kedward & Cooper (1969) showed that a significant proportion of so-called neurotic disorder remitted spontaneously but 15 - 20% persisted to become chronic.

A similar figure has been reported by several researchers for the proportion of acute episodes of depression which go on to become chronic disorders (Robins and Guze, 1972; Paykel et al, 1974; Weissman and Klerman, 1977). Bearing in mind the cumulative nature of this pool of patients it accounts for the frequent misconception amongst GPs that psychiatric morbidity is chronic and intractable despite evidence to the contrary. Dunn and Skuse (1981) following-up a general practice population for 10 years reported that only 1 in 6 female depressives and 1 in 20 males went on to become chronic.

Put another way, Johnson and Mellor (1977) found that of 119 patients diagnosed as depression, 70% recovered within 6 months and a further 10% were markedly improved. This good prognosis at 6 months can reasonably be expected to pertain also at 12 months on the basis of studies done by other researchers. Widmer and Cadoret (1978) examined the outcome of 154 patients diagnosed as "primary depressive disorder" over a mean follow-up period of 6 years. 65% of the sample had only one episode of illness during this time, 26% had two episodes and a further 9% had three episodes or more. The mean duration of an episode was four months with only 13% of episodes lasting longer than two years. This is a profile similar in many respects to that reported in hospital studies. The duration of illness was shorter in primary care, the recovery rate was marginally better and the proportion who relapsed was somewhat smaller but, on the whole, the similarities between the hospital and primary care samples far outweigh the differences.

There is much criticism of the treatment of depressive illness in primary care. Firstly, GPs are accused of not being able to detect depressive disorder and when they do they are criticised either for not treating it at all or treating it subtherapeutically or, worse, treating it with anxiolytics. GPs tend to prescribe in terms of the most predominant symptoms. Where anxiety and depression are mixed a GP tends to resort to an antidepressant if the depression seems more obvious and an anxiolytic if the reverse is true (Downing and Rickels, 1974; Clare and Williams, 1981).

But it is a difficult decision to make. The degree of distress does not appear to influence the decision to prescribe antidepressants but several studies show the presence of sleep disturbance to be an important factor.

Herein lies one of the paradoxes of prescribing in primary care. GPs often maintain that subtherapeutic doses of antidepressants do work and it may well be that one of the changes they bring about is an improvement in sleep patterns. Without well-designed follow-up studies it is difficult to assess the extent to which this alone contributes to improved circumstances and a consequent lifting of mood. The whole question of prescribing habits in primary care is a complex one and psychiatrists would do well to withhold some of their criticism until it is better understood.

Efficacy of Tricyclics in General Practice

Thompson et al (1982) reviewed all the available literature on treatment with tricyclics and were forced to conclude that there were no properly conducted outcome studies of treatment in the primary care setting. They then undertook their own study which illustrated rather well the problems they too then encountered. Starting with 115 carefully selected patients they compared three treatment groups -amitriptyline, L-tryptophan and amitriptyline and tryptophan - with placebo. The treatment groups were all statistically superior to placebo at 6 weeks and 3 months, but by this time almost third of the patients had dropped out of the study. Whilst not affecting the statistical significance of the result this has important practical implications for the GP in his attempts to treat patients. The drop outs were fairly evenly distributed across all groups including the placebo group and for all the usual reasons: slow initial response to treatment, side effects, drug interactions and a dislike of being treated in a pharmacological way for what is experienced as a complex psychosocial condition.

We tackled the problem from a different angle by selecting out depressed patients who had been taking supposedly appropriate doses of tricyclic antidepressants and comparing them with a control group who had received subtherapeutic doses. After one year there was essentially no difference in the proportion still ill in each group but the patients who had been optimally treated had significantly shorter episodes of depression.

So, effective treatment can substantially reduce the period of debility and ill-health. Knowing this, we may feel, as therapists, that treatment is justified. It is more difficult to prove such benefits in terms which will satisfy the cost-effectiveness equation. In weighing-up the balance we also need to know more about the effect of treatment on preventing future relapses.

A very serious consequence of failure to treat effectively, and one which we were unable to address in our own sample due to the infrequency of very severe depression, is the heightened risk of suicide occurring. Recently we have begun to analyse the factors associated with successful suicides that have occurred in Hackney inpatients and we found two features recurring. One is the tendency for doctors to underestimate the severity of depression and the other is the failure to treat effectively by either delays in commencing medication or treating with subtherapeutic doses of antidepressants.

Conclusions

Given that the bulk of depressive disorders are presenting and being treated in the primary care setting and that these patients are being diagnosed more accurately and frequently, does it make any difference in the long run if they are treated with antidepressants? The tentative answers are in the affirmative. We can certainly alter the duration of the illness and alleviate to some extent the experience of depressed mood. More importantly but still unknown are questions about the long-term effects on relapse rates and suicidal behaviour. By comparison with the wealth of information we have about the psychiatric morbidity of hospital patients very little is known about the primary care population. In order to address the issues involved in "failure to treat" we need much more information about:-

The prevalence and nature of depression in primary care

its presentation and identification

natural history

treatment outcomes.

References

1. Brown G.W., Craig T.K.J. and Harris T.O. (1985). Depression: disease or distress? Some epidemiological considerations. Br.J.Psychiat. *147:* 612 - 622.
2. Clare A.W. and Williams P. (1981). Factors leading to psychotropic drug treatment. In: The Misuse of Psychotropic Drugs. London. Gaskell Books.
3. Downing R.W. and Rickels K. (1974). Mixed anxiety and depression: fact or myth? Arch. Gen. Psychiat. *30:* 312 - 317.
4. Dunn G. and Skuse D. (1981). The natural history of depression in general practice: statistical models. Psychol. Med. *11:* 755 - 764.
5. Johnson D.A.W. and Mellor V. (1977). The severity of depression in patients treated in general practice. J of the RCGP *27:* 419 . 422.
6. Kedward H.B. and Cooper B. (1969). Neurotic disorders in urban practice: a three-year follow-up. J of the RCGP *12:* 148 - 163.
7. Paykel E.S., Klerman G.L. and Prusoff B.A. (1974). Prognosis of depression and the endogenous-neurotic distinction. Psychol. Med. *4:* 57 - 64.
8. Robins E. and Guze S. (1972). Classification of affective disorders: the primary-secondary, the endogenous and the neurotic-psychotic concepts. In: Recent Advances in the Psychobiology of the Depressive Illnesses. Publ. Dept. Health, Education & Welfare 70 - 9053.
9. Sireling L.I., Paykel E.S., Freeling P., Rau B.M. and Patel S.P. (1985). Depression in general practice: clinical features and comparison with out-patients. Br. J. Psychiat. *147:* 113 - 118.
10. Thompson J., Rankin H., Ashcroft C.W., Yates C.M. et al (1982). The treatment of depression in general practice. Psychol. Med. *12:* 741 - 751.
11. Weissman M. and Klerman G.L. (1977). The chronic depressive in the community: unrecognised and poorly treated. Comprehensive Psychiat. *18:* 523 - 532.
12. Widmer R B and Cadoret R J (1978). Depression in primary care: changes in pattern of patient visits and complaints during development of depression. J. Family Practice *7:* 293 - 302.

Discussion

Audience: In Cooper's study in Nottingham he observed that for every depressed patient a GP refers to a psychiatrist there may be another 4 or 5 he does not. Could you elaborate on the factors which underlie this selection process?

Clare: Cooper was talking about the overall profile of psychiatric morbidity whereas I have confined my comments to depression. About half of our sample could have been defined as "adjustment disorder", i.e. cases displaying a response to stress that fell short of classical depression and was shortlived. A great many of these turn up and the GP who adopts a "wait and see" attitude handles them very well because invariably time and social manipulation resolve the problems involved. Why some patients come to psychiatrists and others do not depends on the doctor, the patient and the interaction. Some doctors have a very idiosyncratic view of who should be referred. In others it is determined by what the local psychiatric services have to offer, and this varies across the country.

Patients themselves influence the referral system either by a failure to respond to treatment or by indicating that they wish to see a specialist. GPs are more likely to refer psychiatric morbidity associated with gross behavioural disturbance, suicidal threat, or co-existing alcohol and drug abuse. GPs seem better able to pick up depression in women, particularly those of lower socio-economic status. More often undetected are male patients, the very old and very young, so they are under-represented in referrals.

Audience: What difference has the community psychiatric nurse made to referral rates to hospital?

Clare: I do not know. In our areas the CPN is largely involved in the care of the chronic psychiatric population in the community which hardly overlaps at all with the patients we were studying.

TOXICITY IN OVERDOSE

J A Henry
Consultant Physician
National Poisons Unit, Guy's Hospital, London

Hippocrates' time-honoured dictum "primum, non nocere" takes on a new urgency in the context of the recently announced increase in subscriptions to medical defence unions. Since the antidepressant drugs are frequently implicated in deliberate, often fatal, self-poisoning, it is a dictum of particular relevance to those treating depressed patients. However, weighing up the contribution of antidepressant drugs to the therapeutic armamentarium, their major risks - of life-threatening adverse reactions and fatal toxicity - need to be balanced against their benefits in terms of clinical effectiveness. In addressing this problem we have used the Fatal Toxicity Index (Cassidy and Henry, 1987) as a means of estimating the relative hazards or safety of those antidepressant drugs marketed in the U.K. during the years 1975 - 1984.

Tricyclic Antidepressants

Deaths from this group of antidepressants have remained relatively constant over the years 1975 - 1984 (Figure 1).

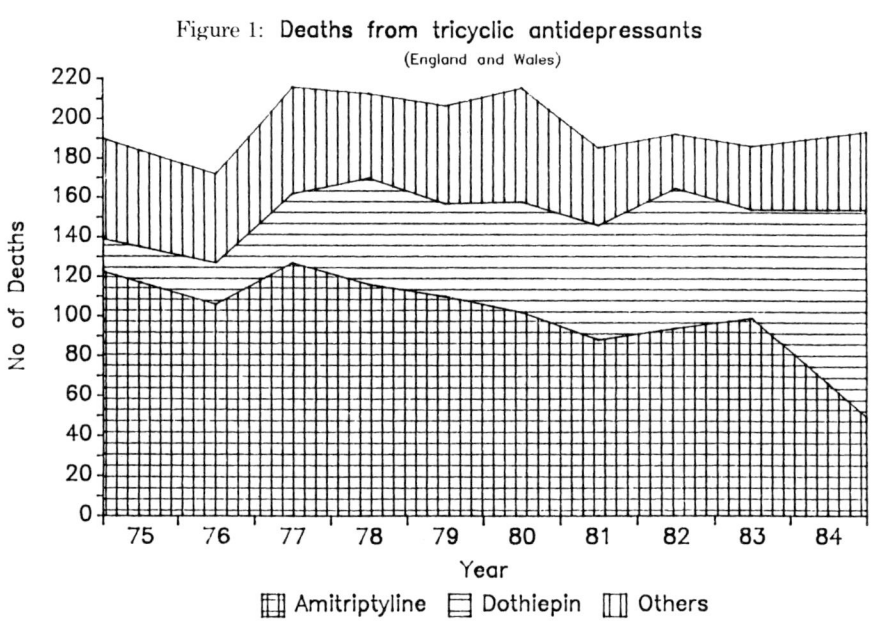

Figure 1: **Deaths from tricyclic antidepressants** (England and Wales)

However, during this time, deaths from amitriptyline have shown a steady decline whilst those from dothiepin have increased. Several factors contribute to the continuing high number of deaths.

The first point is the relationship between the therapeutic and lethal dose ranges. The therapeutic dose range is 1 to 4 mg/kg/day. The lethal dose is in the region of 15 to 20 mg/kg. Thus, death can occur with an overdose of 4 to 20 times the daily dose, which is not a massive amount. Whilst it is possible to survive much larger doses than this it is important to remember that death can occur with a relatively small overdose making it quite easy to kill oneself with these drugs.

The second point is that most deaths (70 - 80%; Crome and Newman, 1979) from tricyclic antidepressant poisoning occur outside hospital. The majority of people who take a tricyclic overdose are deeply depressed and take steps to ensure that they are not found. In general, the people who die from tricyclic antidepressant poisoning are not making a gesture that goes tragically wrong. They intend to die; suicide is one of the hazards of depressive illness, and many patients attempt suicide by overdosing on their medication.

Accidental poisoning in children is another aspect of tricyclic toxicity, numerically quite small, but tragic by proportion. In the period 1974 - 1980 there were 100 deaths from accidental poisoning in children under 5 (Craft, 1983) in England and Wales, which means about 10 to 15 deaths per year. Of the 70% which were attributable to drugs, most resulted from ingestion of tricyclics. So this group of drugs poses a serious problem in small children and great care should be taken when prescribing them to mothers who are depressed and disorganised while trying to cope with the demands of a young family.

Table I
Clinical Features of Tricyclic Poisoning

Sinus Tachycardia
Mydriasis
Coma
QRS prolongation
Hyperreflexia
Convulsions
Cardiac Arrhythmias
Hypotension

The anticholinergic effects produce sinus tachycardia and mild mydriasis. About half of the patients reaching hospital are not comatose, they are conscious. They may be agitated or hallucinating but may quickly lose consciousness. Prolongation of the QRS interval on the electrocardiogram is a characteristic sign and a good index of toxicity. Another interesting clinical feature is that the patient may be hypereflexic, with extensor plantar reflexes and loss of conjugate gaze, a picture which can mimic a stroke. However, the combination of equal, symmetrical, brisk reflexes together with loss of conjugate eye movements is typical of tricyclic antidepressant poisoning. Convulsions are common, as are cardiac arrhythmias and hypotension. On a typical ECG the QRS complex will be somewhat wider than normal but not grossly bizarre. It looks a bit like a bundle branch block which then recovers with time but not necessarily in direct relation to the decline in plasma drug levels. Sometimes the QRS complexes remain wide despite normal plasma levels and this may indicate those people who are likely to have arrhythmias later on.

Mechanism of Fatal Toxicity

Deaths from tricyclic antidepressant overdose are usually due to arrhythmias and/or hypotension. Tricyclic antidepressant toxicity is mainly due to the quinidine-like action of these drugs on cardiac tissue and it is this quinidine-like or membrane-stabilising effect that is ultimately responsible for death (Pentel and Benowitz, 1986).

How does membrane stabilising activity (MSA) cause poisoning? It is the non-specific interaction between membrane lipid bilayers and many lipophilic drugs and chemicals. The drug molecules invade the lipid membrane of the cell and physically interrupt the normal contiguous contact between cells thus spacing them out. In conducting tissue this "stabilises" or slows conduction of impulses, hense its name. Tricyclics have potent MSA which is the property responsible for the profound hypotension, prolongation of QRS complexes and potentially fatal cardiac arrhythmias. Cerebral hypoxia results from both impaired circulation and a direct depression of the respiratory centre which, in turn, causes further central nervous depression and the inevitable death of the patient.

Table II
Management of Tricyclic Poisoning

1. Prevent absorption
   - Gastric lavage
   - Activated charcoal
2. Symptomatic treatment
   - antiarrhythmic drugs
   - anticonvulsants
   - inotropic agents
   - bicarbonate
   - physostigmine
3. Supportive care

Gastric lavage is a traditional step in the acute management of the patient with tricyclic overdose. Whilst currently the subject of some controversy it is, nevertheless, an essential early step for medico-legal reasons and there is no doubt that retrieving large quantities of tablets actually saves lives. Some prefer to give activated charcoal which achieves the same end by absorbing drugs in the stomach if it is given early enough. Again, there is some debate as to its efficacy but it remains an accepted method of preventing drug absorption. I have not included the use of an emetic, because the risk of causing vomiting once the patient has lost consciousness is too great. Once the stomach has been emptied many other drugs have been employed to treat the complications symptomatically (Table II). Sodium bicarbonate is perhaps one of the most useful treatments even in the absence of a metabolic acidosis in that it helps the heart beat more effectively, perhaps as a result of redistribution of the drug due to a pH effect. All the other drugs in Table II have been tried - physostigmine only as a last ditch measure - but the mainstay of treatment and what can ultimately ensure survival is supportive care. Simple, basic, resuscitative measures such as external cardiac massage can sustain life if maintained until the patient recovers or catabolises the drug. This type of poisoning is very non-specific, so provided life can be supported until the drug effects have worn off, and cerebral hypoxia has not occurred, a full recovery can be anticipated.

Monoamine Oxidase Inhibitors (MAOIs)

There are three fundamental problems with this group of drugs:

1. The "cheese" reaction
2. Interaction with tricyclics
3. Toxicity in overdose

The "cheese" reaction, so called because it was first noted in relation to cheese, occurs because some cheeses are rich in tyramine which, as an indirectly acting amine, produces a hypertensive crisis when its breakdown is inhibited. The interaction of MAOIs with tricyclics, when they are taken therapeutically in combination, does not cause a hypertensive reaction, but one similar to the reaction seen in MAOI overdose. Clomipramine is particularly liable to interact with MAOIs in this way.

Overdosage produces a serotoninergic-like syndrome. The symptoms may be initially deceptively mild but rapidly progress over 24 hours to include agitation, tremor, alternating low and high blood pressure, severe muscle spasms, hyperpyrexia and convulsions. It is a very dramatic pattern. The patient sweats profusely, has fixed, dilated pupils, the jaw is rigid and they very often have opisthotonos. It can be confused with tetanus and is mediated at a spinal level. Most curiously, although the half-life of these drugs is just a couple of hours, the reaction builds up over 18 to 24 hours, the patient gradually deteriorating despite undetectable plasma drug levels.

Illustrative Case History: Tricyclic/MAOI Interaction

Patient: Female - aged 40 years.

Treatment: Tranylcypromine and trifluoperazine overdose.

Summary: After 9 hours the patient was flushed, agitated and shivering. By the 10th hour she had trismus and was unable to speak. Opisthotonos was observed, she was sweating profusely, had fixed, dilated pupils, pulse 140 beats/minute, blood pressure 170/100 and an axillary temperature of 38°C. There was no response to the administration of diazepam. When the rectal temperature continued rising to 41°C she was intubated and ventilated. Paralysis was initially achieved using succinylcholine and then maintained with pancuronium. This single step was responsible for reducing her temperature to normal over the course of the next 10 hours.

This pattern occurs commonly after an MAOI overdose, it is a very dramatic presentation and not easy to recognise unless one has prior experience of the condition. Despite fully active heat-losing mechanisms the temperature continues to rise, heat being generated by the severe muscle spasm. Unless intervention is rapid the patient dies of heatstroke which denatures the body's proteins. Once muscle relaxation is achieved the body's temperature regulation mechanisms are able to cope, the temperature starts to fall and recovery can be expected.

Second Generation Antidepressants

I am not going to go into the newer antidepressants in detail except to say they have different chemical structures, they have differing modes of action and, in general, their toxicity is lower. There are, by and large, few symptoms from overdoses of the newer drugs.

Mortality Data

We have used national mortality statistics and prescription data to compile fatal toxicity indices (FTIs) of the currently available antidepressant drugs in order to assess their comparative safety from an epidemiological standpoint (Cassidy and Henry, 1987). There are pros and cons in using mortality data which should be borne in mind when interpreting calculations based upon them. Mortality indicates the most serious toxicity, it is numerically discrete and it provides a clearly definable end point. For all these reasons it is an attractive statistic. On the other hand the data are susceptible to several sources of error and inaccuracy. It is not always easy from the material available to deduce accurate diagnoses. Death certificates are only as accurate as the physician recording the details. By collecting large series of figures it is hoped that errors and misdiagnoses either cancel each other out or become insignificant. The other problem with mortality data is that it needs to be interpreted against a background of the availability of each drug in the community. In the U.K. this can be estimated using records collated by the National Health Service of the number of prescriptions issued. This fails to take into account private prescriptions but overall this is a very small source of bias. Other indices used include estimations of the number of tablets prescribed or the quantity (kg) of each drug used. Whichever of these methods is used, similar results are produced.

We used OPCS mortality data for 1975 - 1984 for England and

Wales combined with the Registrar General's data for the same period for Scotland, and for Prescription data 1975 - 84 for England, Scotland and Wales we used the NHS data. The null hypothesis was tested using a chi-squared test.

The Fatal Toxicity Index (FTI)

Figure 2

Toxicity of Major Groups of Antidepressants 1974 - 84

Drug Group	Number of Deaths	Deaths per 10^6 Prescriptions
Monoamine Oxidase Inhibitors	42	26.7
Tricyclic Antidepressants (1970 and before)	2384	38.5 ***
Tricyclic and other Antidepressants (1974 and after)	125	13.0 ***
(All Antidepressants	2551	34.9)***

*** Different from all Antidepressants ($P < 0.001$)

Figure 2 shows a comparison of the toxicity of the major groups of antidepressants before 1970 and after 1974. The total number of deaths was 2551 which gave an overall 34.9% deaths per million prescriptions as a baseline for comparison of each individual group of drugs. The early tricyclics as a group are significantly worse ($p<0.001$) than the group of all antidepressants. MAOIs do not attain statistical significance because of the small number of deaths in that group.

Looking specifically at the tricyclics (Figure 3) these are ranked according to the number of deaths per million scripts. Desipramine, dothiepin and amitriptyline are all high on the list and exceed the mean FTI for all antidepressants. Imipramine is statistically a safer drug but this should be interpreted with caution since about 15% of imipramine scripts are for nocturnal eneuresis in children which tends to bias the figure and give a false sense of safety. Clomipramine, imipramine, iprindole, protriptyline and trimipramine all had a significantly lower FTI than the mean of all antidepressants which suggests a possible safety advantage of these 5 drugs.

Figure 3
Tricyclic Antidepressants

Drug	Number of Deaths	Deaths per 10^6 Prescriptions
Dibenzepin	4	157.5 **
Desipramine	13	80.2 **
Dothiepin	533	50.0 ***
Amitriptyline	1181	46.5 ***
Nortriptyline	57	39.2 NS
Doxepin	102	31.3 NS
Imipramine	278	28.4 ***
Trimipramine	155	27.6 **
Opipramol	2	21.8 NS
Clomipramine	51	11.1 ***
Protriptyline	6	10.3 **
Iprindole	2	7.8 **
(All Antidepressants	2551	34.9 -)

*** $P < 0.001$]
** $P < 0.01$] From All Antidepressants
* $P < 0.05$]

Figure 4
Monoamine Oxidase Inhibitors

Drug	Number of Deaths	Deaths per 10^6 Prescriptions
Tranylcypromine	15	58.1 NS
Phenylzine	24	22.8 *
Isocarboxazid	3	12.8 *
Iproniazid	0	0.0 NS
(All Antidepressants	2551	34.9 -)

* $P < 0.05$ From All Antidepressants

The next group of drugs are the MAOIs (Figure 4) and the statistical significances are weak because of the smaller number involved, although my suspicion is that there are more deaths from MAOIs which are not recognised. People come in to hospital with bizarre hyperthermic syndromes which are misdiagnosed as, say, heatstroke or fulminating infection. Another problem is that the figures refer to "single drug only" deaths, while some MAOIs are prescribed in combined formulations.

Figure 5
Antidepressants Introduced After 1973

Drug	Number of Deaths		Deaths per 10^6 Prescriptions
	Observed	Expected	
Maprotiline	83	77	37.6 NS
Trazodone	6	15	13.6 *
Viloxazine	2	7.4	9.4 *
Butriptyline	1	4.7	7.5 NS
Mianserin	30	187	5.6 ***
Nomifensine	3	42	2.5 ***
Lofepramine	0	3.7	0.0 NS
(All Antidepressants	2551	—	34.9 -)

*** $P < 0.001$]
* $P < 0.05$] From All Antidepressants

Much interest is now focused on the newer antidepressants. With the exception of maprotiline which approximates the tricyclics chemically, structually and in its FTI, all the others in this group (Figure 5) have much lower FTIs, suggesting that progress has been made in producing drugs which are less toxic. The safety of mianserin and nomifensine (now withdrawn) in overdose has a strong statistical significance, but nomifensine has caused a further 25 deaths from haemolytic anaemias and allergies which are outside the scope of the FTI. How some of the newer antidepressants will fare remains to be seen. This kind of analysis is an ongoing exercise and the figures need updating from time to time as new data become available.

Conclusion

These figures invite further consideration and provide an approach to more rational prescribing. Amitriptyline and several related tricyclics have higher fatal toxicity indices than the MAOIs which are, in turn, more toxic that a number of newer antidepressants. Among the drugs introduced since 1973, all have a favourable toxicity profile except maprotiline. If the newer drugs have as good a record of clinical effectiveness combined with their apparent lower potential to cause fatal poisoning when taken in overdose, serious consideration should be given to preferentially prescribing the newer drugs, especially in situations where suicidal overdose is a possibility.

References

1. Cassidy S., Henry J. (1987). Fatal toxicity of antidepressants in overdose. British Medical Journal *295*, 1021 - 1024.
2. Craft A.W. (1983). Circumstances surrounding deaths from accidental poisoning 1974 - 1980. Archives of Disease in Childhood *58*. 544 - 546.
3. Crome P., Newman B. (1979). Fatal tricyclic antidepressant poisoning. Journal of Royal Society of Medicine *72*, 649 - 653.
4. Pentel P.R., Benowitz N.L. (1986). Tricyclic antidepressant poisoning: management of arrhythmias. Medical Toxicology *1*, 101 - 121.

Discussion

Audience: Do you think MAOIs should be banned?

Henry: I am against banning drugs. We should be taught to use them properly and to balance benefits against risks. Some people will respond quite dramatically to MAOIs when no other drug will work so it would be unfair to take them off the market altogether. There are new MAOIs being developed which will have a more selective mode of action but until they are available we should retain the original ones.

Audience: Reviewing the ADRs mentioned by Leonard in fatalities per million and combining these with the overdose figures presented here, all tricyclics appear to be very bad drugs and the newer drugs appear to be good from a fatality perspective. Would you agree?

Henry: Yes, by and large, most of the data support the same conclusions.

Audience: Are your prescription numbers based on both GP and hospital scripts?

Henry: National Health Service pharmacy scripts only are included - in other words GP prescriptions and not hospital or private scripts.

REPORTING THE RISKS

C Speirs
Lecturer in Toxicology
Hammersmith Hospital, London.

Beyond the controlled clinical trial setting the reporting of adverse reactions to drugs (ADRs) in "real life" poses many problems, not least of which is the attention of the media. Bad news about drugs **is** news, good news is not worth reporting. As doctors we need to take a measured view of the situation and look at ADR monitoring in the context of drug development because the full risk/benefit ratio can only be revealed when the drug is on the market.

Before considering ADR monitoring in more detail it is always instructive to review the development strategy behind a drug. Some of the advantages claimed for newer antidepressants in terms of minimised sedation, for example, which theoretically reduces the potential for car accidents, can be anticipated from the original studies of animal pharmacology. Prediction of problems such as teratogenicity, mutagenicity and carcinogenesis might also stem from pre-clinical work. Any hint of a problem during drug development directs attention into these specific areas when the drug is marketed. Post-marketing surveillance has thus to be seen in context against a background of animal and human pharmacology, pharmacokinetics and clinical trials and their implications for experience in the "real world". Efficacy in comparison to placebo may then be established more clearly. The role of the drug within the therapeutic armamentarium is something that may take years to evolve. Post-marketing surveillance is the final aspect of drug development and demands an equally rigorous approach if excessive pharmacological reactions beyond the prime activity of the drug are to be identified. Toxic effects such as hepatitis may occur, or idiosyncratic reactions or unexpected differences between humans and animals in immunological reactions or metabolic processes.

Adverse reactions are divided into the predictable (type A) and unpredictable (type B) reactions and we should perhaps add a further (type C) reaction which is not in the textbooks - the reactions which might reasonably have been predicted had all prior information about the drug been carefully analysed. The exaggerated effects of a preparation in the elderly, for example, and the differences in dosage. Many so-called surprises could be avoided if basic extrapolations such as these were made. Dosage is a fundamental aspect of drug development since the administration of a higher dosage than necessary only serves to increase the potential for unwanted side effects developing.

What then, is the aim of post-marketing surveillance (PMS)? Most attention is focussed on the rare, unexpected and serious type B idiosyncratic adverse reactions. The emergence of these has been responsible for the withdrawal of several antidepressant preparations. But the aim is also to look for the natural or "real world" incidence of type A adverse reactions. The fatal toxicity index described by Henry (Henry and Cassidy, op cit.) demonstrates mortality from suicide very clearly. Morbidity in terms of what is often (erroneously) dismissed as trivial events is much more difficult to quantify accurately. Clinical trials are not ideal because they are limited by patient selection, by the duration of exposure to treatment and the relatively small numbers of patients involved. PMS tries to redress some of these shortcomings and tends to concentrate more on the idiosyncratic ADRs which have not been predicted.

The different methods of PMS can be roughly divided into the collection of spontaneous reports which are non-systematic and include reports from the medical literature and systematic reports as pioneered by the yellow card system in the U.K. An obvious but very basic problem with this approach is one of validity. Not all reports are necessarily true instances of ADRs. Presumably the reports made in the literature can be reliably attributed to ADRs but with yellow cards and spontaneous reports the reliability of the information can be very variable and subjective. Serendipity often dictates whether a doctor is sufficiently moved to report a reaction that has come to his attention - or an insistent patient who has read ADR publicity.

The Boston Collaborative Drug Surveillance Programme which has proved to be expensive and difficult to establish is not generally applicable. Although huge numbers of patients were included in this monitoring attempt, about half a million case records were searched, there was still not enough patients in each drug category to detect idiosyncratic reactions with any degree of confidence. Such studies can, however, produce interesting information concerning actual prescribing habits in their catchment area and of previously unsuspected drug interactions.

Epidemiological surveys provide a way of systematically studying ADRs using vital statistics, following cohorts of patients or retrospectively doing case control studies. What is generated by the spontaneous report method of collecting data is a signal and not scientific fact. Epidemiological studies are the natural sequel to the unsystematic spontaneous report and carry more weight in establishing scientific fact because they increase certainty, albeit without proof. The linking of a drug to an adverse reaction often proceeds in this way but the causality of the association has to be established using more rigorous methods.

One such system is the Prescription Event Monitoring system developed in Southampton in which prescriptions (particularly those for new drugs) are linked to any **event** that might occur. Unfortunately there is, as yet, little information on the newer antidepressants to illustrate the following points because experience with these drugs is still limited.

The yellow card system is an old type of spontaneous reporting system in which doctors are asked to report "any untoward condition in the patient which might be the result of drug treatment" (Sir Derek Dunlop, May 1966 in a letter to all doctors). This refers essentially to suspected ADRs. The data has to be collected in such a way that information is not inadvertently duplicated which is difficult enough but is not the main pitfall with this approach. The basic difficulty with this system is with information processing. The first step in interpretation of spontaneously reported data is by "eyeballing", the efficiency of which depends very much on the experience and sensitivity of the interpreter. The signal is raised that a drug is associated with a particular problem then the next step is to establish a direct link before definitive action can be taken.

To illustrate the system in practise I shall draw on the familiar example of zimelidine, an antidepressant now withdrawn from the market. A serotonin re-uptake inhibitor, zimelidine had been shown in clinical trials to be relatively free of central anticholinergic side effects. Its release onto the market in Sweden in March 1982 was soon followed by reports of suspected ADRs. A flu-like illness 7 - 14 days after commencing treatment was reported several times. This was accompanied by a high fever, general malaise, arthralgia, headache, nausea and occasionally raised liver transminases. The reports were mainly from GPs. Two patients were admitted to hospital with aseptic meningitis. Later that year adverse reaction assessors in the Swedish service (SADRAC) noticed a case of polyradiculitis associated with drug treatment. When the company was contacted they were able to confirm that one case of ascending myelitis had in fact occurred during clinical trials in 1979. Being a very rare disease it was assumed to have arisen by chance and there was no question of trying to establish causality. These cases were reported by SADRAC in an effort to ellicit further reports through publicity and, sure enough, 8 further reports followed. The annual incidence of Guillaine Barre syndrome is 2.5 cases per 100,000 population. Zimelidine exposure was estimated at 14,000 patient years which should have produced only a third of the cases reported. Neurological opinion was satisfied that 6 patients definitely had Guillaine Barre syndrome and three further cases were "possibles". Causality was thus demonstrated and the drug subsequently withdrawn.

But why in fact should it have been withdrawn? How can these adverse reaction findings be adequately weighed against the favourable aspects of the drug in any meaningful sort of way? One imagines a scientific balancing act being rigorously performed by anonymous government officials intent on protecting the patient's best interests but what in fact happens is rather different. It is a somewhat crude consideration influenced partly by the law and partly by the emotive effect of the media. In the case of zimelidine the company responsible chose to withdraw the drug on the professional opinion of their lawyers that the ensuing liability for damages would be unsustainable. Judgement was thus a combination of judicial opinion and public perception that 9 neurological problems per 14,000 patient years of drug use outweighed the clinical advantages of the drug. And this is a fairly typical sequence of events in an ADR.

Using the spontaneous reporting system it is possible to build up a profile of ADR reporting. The suspected ADRs for antidepressants when grouped together into organ systems give a quick, simple way of monitoring suspicious signals. For example, in the skin category, it can be seen that protriptyline causes photodermatitis whereas the other drugs do not. Imipramine is associated with urticaria. The lack of accompanying prescribing data, however, limits the conclusions which can be drawn from these observations. In order to compare ADRs in a meaningful way the indications and efficacy of the drugs in question should also be taken into account. In rheumatology, gold and penicillamine are retained in clinical practise despite considerable problems with ADRs but their use is restricted to the treatment of very ill patients for whom the potential benefits outweigh the possible toxicity. Several of the now-banned anti-inflammatories carried less risk of harm, despite publicity to the contrary, but were considered to be unacceptable because their use was over a much wider spectrum of less severe disease. Adequate prescription data is always difficult to obtain but the more widespread use of computerisation should aid rapid access to data in the future.

We also need to take account of bias in the reporting of ADRs. Phenylbutazone and oxyphenbutazone were withdrawn due to haematological problems, being responsible for half of all aplastic anaemias in this country in the late 60's and early 70's. And yet the ADR reporting rate per million scripts was in fact far lower for these toxic drugs than for the less toxic ones which have been reported 100 times more frequently. Herein lies a major source of bias in that there is an enormously greater reporting rate for new drugs as opposed to established ones with a known spectrum of side effects. New drugs are always disadvantaged in overall reporting rates. Reporting itself is a highly selective, subjective procedure depending on an interaction of variables between doctor, patient and drug. Reports in journals often provoke a flurry of interest in a drug and result in increased ADR reporting. The effects of media publicity, as mentioned earlier, can be potent. Changing drug usage is another factor to be taken into account. If MAOIs are used to treat a different group of depressed patients than tricyclic antidepressants then again the ADRs will not be directly comparable albeit not necessarily invalid. Selective marketing of a drug also results in an altered pattern of ADR reporting.

Prescription Event Monitoring

Prescription event monitoring, by providing an accurate denominator and numerator, addresses some of the problems with the other survey methods. This method was pioneered in the U.K. by Professor Inman's group in Southampton. The scale of the operation is daunting with prescriptions for new drugs extracted at the rate of 0.5 million scripts per year which are then processed at the Drug Surveillance Research Unit (fig 1).

Figure 1: Phase I

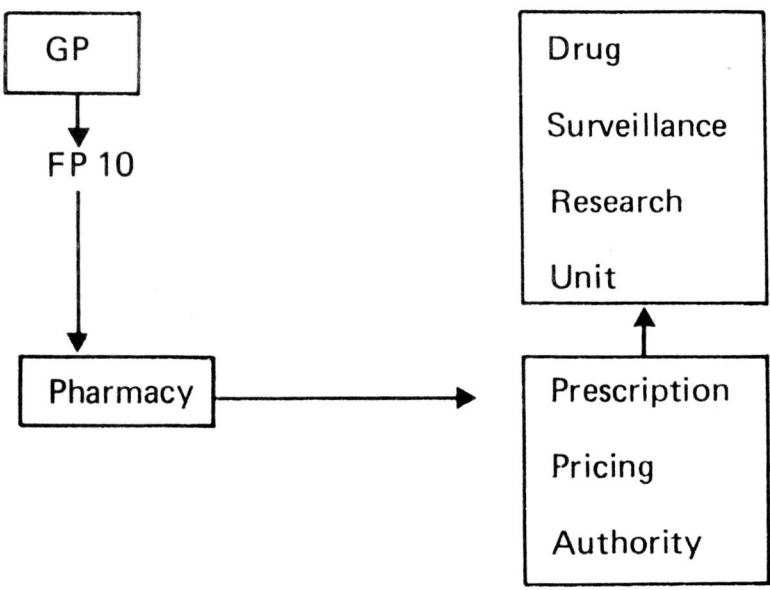

Approximately 120,000 requests for event reporting (fig 2) have been sent to doctors on one specific drug. The scale is thus somewhat unwieldy but it has the great advantage of providing a very clear denominator in the patients identified. The numerator, or event, which may or may not be causally linked to the drug is defined broadly as "any new diagnosis, referral or admission, unexpected improvement or change of treatment".

Figure 2: Questions for G.P.

1. Any "events" (including reason for stopping drug) since start of treatment?
2. Referral to hospital?
3. N.H.S. No. and date of birth?

An "event" is any new diagnosis, accident, unexpected deterioration or improvement, cause of death, suspected ADR etc.

The analysis of events after prescriptions is always a comparison (fig 3) either to a background risk of the event occurring or to the incidence found with other drugs. Alternatively, the number of events occurring during the after treatment can be compared.

Figure 3: Analysis of data

1. **Compare event-profiles**
   a. Other P.E.M. drugs
   b. ADR experience
   c. Morbidity and mortality statistics
2. **Further action**
   a. More-detailed follow-up of individual patients
   b. Ad hoc studies

Ultimately, the objective is to obtain comparative data between different drugs of the same therapeutic class derived from their use in the "real world" of clinical medicine. Systems such as the one in operation at the DSRU at Southampton are now capable of achieving this objective. The first obstacle lies in obtaining sufficient numbers of reports - in a comparison of mianserin with amitriptyline for example some 180,000 reports have been solicited from GPs. Then their are problems in interpretation of the data bearing in mind the various sources of bias referred to earlier. Nevertheless, as Rothschild has said, "comparisons, far from being odious, are the best antidote to panic".

DISCUSSION

Audience: Remembering back to such episodes as the thalidomide tragedy and the "cheese reactions", it still seems to take just as long to alert doctors to a serious ADR despite the numbers of people involved in monitoring.

Speirs: I agree, time is of the essence. The advantages of the yellow card system include its potential to reach every patient and every doctor and its availability for immediate scanning. As I showed with zimeldine this is the quickest way of finding something which is quite unusual. With the other system, which has a careful numerator and denominator, it cannot produce results quite so quickly but is more definitive. There is no question of one system replacing another. When comparing an established drug such as amitriptyline with the newer drugs, there are clinical trial side effects profiles and suicide data to go on, but no information about the effects occurring with normal clinical use. Comparisons like this can be very helpful, but they do take time. PEM's most useful function may, in fact, be to show a reduced risk with some drugs.

Bridges: Perhaps we should be more selective in our use of antidepressants. General practitioners could prescribe the newer antidepressants because they are safer and a psychiatrist would have access to a much wider range of drugs to deal with the more persistent and severe depressions. It might thus be possible to avoid such extensive use of the tricyclics. Would you agree Tony?

Clare: Should GPs be using antidepressants at all? There is no consensus about this among psychiatrists. Anthony Mann at the Royal Free Hospital argues very strongly that antidepressants are underused in primary care with severe depressions often being treated, inappropriately, with anxiolytics. Others feel that antidepressants should be very rarely used in general practice for all the reasons we have been discussing today.

If 2,200 general practitioners are using anxiolytics in situations where psychiatrists would use antidepressants, there must be a reason. As a group of drugs they are much less toxic than the antidepressants and if they produce sedation and some relief of anxiety, which consequently lead to a lifting of mood, without nasty side effects, then this is why they are preferred. You were saying, Paul, that perhaps GPs should be encouraged to use the newer antidepressants. I think this is beginning to happen in practise and that amitriptyline and imipramine are decreasing in use. Is this right?

Henry: They are still widely used, but it seems that dothiepin is taking some of the market from amitriptyline.

Clare: That is interesting. Despite all the scientific evidence to the contrary it confirms my impression that many clinicians still feel the older tricyclics are more effective.

Bridges: Yes, and what made a big impression on me from this morning's session was the very high mortality associated with dothiepin which otherwise appears to be a reasonable tricyclic.

Henry: One of the things which concerns me is the way in which a drug is presented to a patient. When prescribing one of the older drugs the doctor warns the patient that the drug will not work for 3 weeks, it may cause drowsiness and a dry mouth but that it is important to persevere with it. With one of the new drugs which has very few side effects, the doctor simply tells the patient to take this and come back in 4 weeks. It may well be that we counsel patients differently and that this interaction with the patient influences compliance and the effectiveness of the drug. This is an aspect which is outside the realms of clinical trial data.

Clare: In our research unit we encourage general practitioners to prescribe the tricyclics in exactly the way you have described. I suspect it is as you say - with the newer drugs we relax and confidently assure the patient, in response to their questions, that these new drugs have none of the side effects of the older ones. I wonder to what extent the "pre-marketing advice" affects the "post-marketing return".

Henry: If you have a feeling of concern or of seriousness when you are instructing the patient then, at some level, this will be perceived and will determine the patient's attitude towards the drug.

Clare: Certainly that is what we are encouraged to do.

Henry: But by doing so we alter their compliance. This is a very big area and one that has not been studied.

Speirs: It is certainly a way in which spontaneous reporting could be very biased, depending on the type of advice that is given to patients and it is exactly the situation where you really need something like an event monitoring system.

Clare: In the Newcastle trial that I referred to a standard package of advice was given to patients because of the double-blind nature of the study and there was quite a high adverse reaction reporting rate in the placebo group as well.

Speirs: At Southampton the PEM group are undertaking a very big study of mianserin and amitriptyline. So far they have had 100,000 prescriptions and 20,000 replies from doctors and they are analysing the ADRs. The original intention was to look at mianserin blood dyscrasias, but what is showing up with overwhelming frequency are the cardiovascular side effects of amitriptyline.

There also seems to be a higher reporting rate for blood dyscrasias with amitriptyline than was anticipated. All drugs need to be compared in this carefully matched way.

Clare: We seem to be very much better at monitoring the risks than the benefits. If there were two drugs and drug "A" was a better drug than drug "B" then patients might be prepared to put up with all manner of side effects, which takes me back to the question of establishing the **benefits** of these drugs in primary care - not just the risks. I have always been impressed by the attempts to monitor risks and side effects but is it not a much more difficult task to demonstrate the benefits?

How do you weigh up the data I gave you today, for example, showing that antidepressants in primary care shorten the duration of a depressive episode against the various, rather grim-looking statistics about suicide and ADRs.

I do not know the answer other than to painstakingly establish efficacy of drug use with or without associated psychotherapy. It is a much more complex and challenging task than it appears.

Speirs: The problem is even wider than that. If I understand it correctly, it look as though mianserin saved 157 people who would have died against 30 who did. How do you balance that against the increased problems with blood dyscrasias? The common theme that comes through is that judgement is based on the public perception of risk.

Henry: It is not just public perception. It is also the CSM's perceived role which influences us. They see their role as simply drug safety, and are not interested in drug overdose. When we show them our data they are more concerned about the person who has died from a blood dyscrasia than the ones who have died from overdose.

Speirs: But is it really up to the central authority or up to us as doctors to examine why the patient has died? That is a matter between the doctor and the patient and the central authority act more as a buffer, as an explanatory body.

Audience: The point that Dr Henry makes that the CSM is interested only in therapeutic doses and take no responsibility for overdosage is a very relevant one and this attitude is quite shortsighted where antidepressants are concerned.

Speirs: Most definitions of adverse reactions exclude deaths from overdose or abuse.

Clare: You may well find a far higher rate of overdosage for amitriptyline than for, say, mianserin, but how can you be sure that the two populations of patients were the same? Traditional teaching has always been that in severe depressive illness the drug of choice was the established "potent" tricyclic antidepressant. When you are treating, for example, a depression associated with physical disease, then you are much more likely to use one of the newer antidepressants.

Bridges: But not in adequate doses, so the patient is taking a continuous risk without any benefit at all.

Audience: One of the interesting points to come out of the study mentioned by Dr Speirs on mianserin versus amitriptyline, is that mianserin seems to be selectively prescribed to the terminally ill, the very old and those with concomitant disease, cardiovascular disease in particular. This brings us back to Professor Clare's point that such selective prescribing to a group with a very high risk of death from physical disease, but not such a high suicide risk, biases the between-drug comparison.

Speirs: All studies contained some sort of bias and in the final analysis you have to decide whether this is sufficiently strong to nullify the tentative conclusions you would have drawn.

LIST OF DELEGATES

ALANI A A — *Poole*
ASHFORD J J — *Southampton*
BARANIECKA V T — *Ashford*
BENSTEAD S — *Ashead*
BLACK A A — *London*
BRADLEY J J — *London*
CHONG T C — *Brighton*
DAWES P — *Sandwich*
DAWLING S — *London*
DAWISHA A I — *Chatham*
DEVAKUMAR V C — *Bacup*
DOMINIAN J — *London*
EARL R — *Nottingham*
FRANKLIN R A — *Poole*
GALLIMORE G R — *Dorchester*
GOONATILLEKE M D A P — *Waterloo*
HERNANDEZ M — *Whitchurch*
HOLLAND P — *Alton*
JESINGER D — *Southampton*
KAPUGE R A — *Kings Lynn*
KIDD G T B — *Chertsey*
LINTNER B — *Charmouth*
MAJID A — *Middlesbrough*
McBRYDE H — *Devizes*
MULLIN J M — *Willerby*
NOSHAD H — *London*
OXBY L — *London*
PHILLIPS W S — *Brentford*
PIEKE R A — *Netherlands*
PINDER R M — *Netherlands*
POYNTON A M — *London*
RASIAH N J — *Epsom*
REZA H — *Fareham*
RICHARDSON M W T — *Cambridge*
ROSE L — *London*
SAHA B N — *Woking*
SAMUEL G — *Petersfield*

SENIOR D — *Willerby*
TARRY J — *Durham*
THOMAS P M — *Carmarthen*
THOMAS S M — *Comberton*
THOMSON M E — *London*
TIMMS P W — *London*
TOWNSEND A — *High Wycombe*
VERMA H M — *Welshpool*
WAGON R — *Blakeney*
WATKIN J H *Epsom*
WHITE J H McN — *Scunthorpe*
WONNACOTT S — *Southampton*